too young
for a
heart
attack

Stu Segal
with Dr. Ian J. Molk

This book is not intended as a substitute for the medical advice of physicians or healthcare professionals. The reader should regularly consult a physician in matters relating to his/her health, and particularly with respect to any symptoms that may require diagnosis or medical attention. The contents of this book represent the experiences, observations, and opinions of Stu Segal, who is not a licensed physician.

ACKNOWLEDGEMENTS

Stephen H. Segal
Editing — Cover Design — Book Design

For their invaluable assistance with this book,
Karen Hohe
Frank P. Beninato, Jr.
Rashmika

DEDICATION

To the many people who helped my recovery over the years,
my family, my friends, my colleagues. For their love and support.
For their friendship and camaraderie. And for enduring, even
encouraging, the obsessions that make my life worth living.

For Barb, Colleen, Dave, Farah, Jimmy, Kathy, Mike, Natalie,
Rashmi, Sammi, Sharon, Stacy, Stephen, Tom and Tony

And to the best physicians anyone could ever hope for.
Their outstanding care and counsel has helped me live
long enough, and well enough, to share this story with you.

My heartfelt thanks to:
Dr. Austin Gerber, D.O., General Practice—Pleasantville, NJ
Dr. David George, D.O., General Practice—Moscow, PA
Dr. Jacob Levin, M.D., Cardiology—Somers Point, NJ
Dr. Marc Mayer, D.O., General Practice—Iselin, NJ
Dr. Mitch Mayer, D.O., General Practice—Iselin, NJ
Dr. Ian J. Molk, M.D., Cardiology—Edison, NJ
Dr. Fred Winter, D.D.S—Metuchen, NJ

Contents

Introduction

I had a heart attack, out of the blue, at age 37. It was serious—serious enough to put me out of work for six months, serious enough to change the rest of my life in ways I couldn't imagine.

It's been 26 years since the heart attack. I have lived, loved, laughed—in spite of the heart attack. Or is it because of the heart attack? Hard to say, but over time it awakened my desire to live and revealed my love of life. It gave me the motivation to stop my unhealthy behaviors, the eating, the smoking, the stressing . . . the behaviors that surely precipitated the crisis.

Prior to the heart attack I never truly recognized the risks of these behaviors. I was thin and had always been thin. I didn't need to exercise or watch what I ate to stay that way. And you know, thin is healthy—just ask anyone.

Once a year an unsuspecting Girl Scout hit the jackpot when she rang our doorbell—I had calculated exactly how many boxes of Thin Mints would fit in our freezer. Once the wide-eyed Scout left with my order, I would begin a mission to eat everything in the freezer before she came back weeks later with cases of cookies. And then I would eat my way through a mountain of chocolaty sugary Thin Mints.

My diet included absolutely no vegetables—if it was green, it wasn't going in my mouth. I loved anything sugary—Frosted Flakes, Pop Tarts, Boston cream pie, Tastykakes. And let's not forget Italian salami, capicola, steaks . . . and hot pastrami sandwiches, calzones, strombolis. Reading in bed at night, I always had candy bars and milk. I loved going to motorcycle rallies—where else could I pull the pork right off a roasted pig, or find racks of barbecued ribs, all juicy and dripping fat? A beer truck with flowing taps yards away. Never any asparagus or broccoli here!

And I smoked. Actually I smoked a lot, two packs a day, and had been smoking for over 20 years. At one time I played a lot of tennis—two mornings a week, plus team tennis, plus tournaments, and lots of practice. Except when in actual tournament play, I smoked while playing—running around the court with a cigarette hanging out of my mouth! I started and ended every day with a cigarette. I knew it was harmful, but figured it wouldn't hurt me, not until I was older . . . and I planned to stop . . . someday . . . before it was too late.

Whether it was what I ate, or smoked, or stressed over, there was no moderation—stuffing the freezer with a years supply of cookies seemed perfectly normal to me. When I liked something, I really liked it; and when I didn't, I avoided it like the plague. Unfortunately, allowing my indulgences (bad diet, smoking, stress) and avoiding my dislikes (exercise, healthy eating) was the perfect formula for a heart attack. Which left me with a damaged heart, forevermore.

Nearly three decades later I can tell you I have lived an amazing life, though in the aftermath of the heart attack I believed it was destined to be an unfulfilling life, a life of restrictions, the life of a cardiac cripple. It has not been without adversity, conflict, depression and setbacks . . . but in the end I beat the odds. I have lived a life many would envy—seeing my children flourish, my career advance, my personal relationships blossom.

This is the story of my journey from the depths of doubt, doubt that I could live, or live fully, to the summit of a life well-lived. From a reckless personal lifestyle which damaged my health, nearly stopped my heart, to an effective, satisfying way of life which halted the advance of heart disease and improved my overall health and well-being. More than just my story, I want to share with you some of the thought processes, techniques and tactics that helped change my life, that put me on the path to better health . . . and that I hope will put you on that same path.

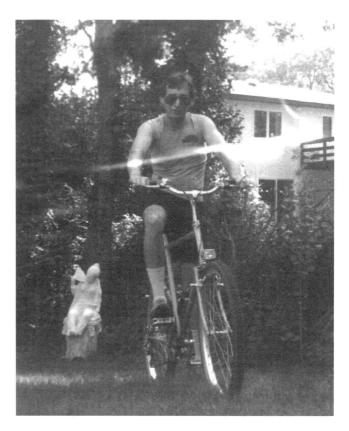

"And you know, thin is healthy—just ask anyone."

part one
heart attack

Will I Live?

It was a perfect day, with an azure sky of deepest summer. And it was the day of the biggest biker event in the state—drag races, custom show, swap meet, rock 'n roll. Thousands of bikes expected. Kathy and the kids were busy; my plan was to meet friends, enjoy the 60 mile ride to the meet, and spend the day looking at bikes and races. Then I was going to head home to a Father's Day dinner.

We left mid-morning, and as we rode to the rally the temperature kept rising. By early afternoon it was in the mid 90s, and sweltering. We spent the day outside, looking at custom bikes, listening to music, perusing the swap meet, and checking out whatever outrageous goings-on we came upon. Midday I had the kind of lunch you could always find at these events, a dripping pulled pork sandwich and a beer.

I was feeling good when we mounted our bikes to head home mid-afternoon. I fired up my bike, was sitting there, engine rumbling, warming up—and there was a cloudburst. We were drenched—from sunny and 90 degrees, to being drenched with freezing rain in an instant! It stopped in a few minutes, and we rode out, the sun drying us as the temperature shot back up into the 90s. Riding along, comfy, warm, dried out . . . then it happened again, drenched with a freezing rain. None of this really bothered me at the time—heat and cold, dry and wet, it's all part of motorcycling. Overall, I thought, a great day.

I got home, took a relaxing shower, and was hanging around the house waiting for dinner. Perhaps an hour later I started to feel hot, and I mean very hot. The sweat was literally dripping off me, my T-shirt was drenched. And I had this pain between my shoulder blades which kept getting worse and worse.

I became so hot that I eventually went outside, started the car, and put the air conditioner on full blast, aimed at me. The pain between my shoulder blades had intensified; I can only describe it as what it must feel like if someone was stabbing you in the back, driving a knife directly between your shoulder blades and through to your heart (it was not, by the way, a crushing pain in the chest, radiating down the arms). I knew something was wrong, but given the lack of what I thought were the traditional symptoms, I certainly didn't think it was a heart attack.

Kathy came out, looked at me, and said "We're going to the hospital"—I was beyond arguing as she started the car. I didn't even notice her driving, which had been the object of both mirth and fear over the years.

This was the day I found out that you don't always have to wait your turn in the emergency room. Once someone said, "chest pain" a flurry of activity began. I was thrown on a gurney, tubes were hooked up to me, people put things in my mouth, electrodes were glued to my chest, I was given shots.

There was an ER doctor, there were nurses, they were running around doing things. My head felt like it was going to explode (I later learned about nitroglycerin). With all the running around, there was one thing that didn't change—the horrible pain, it still felt like someone was driving a knife into my back, right between my shoulder blades. And I was becoming concerned; it seemed they couldn't stop the pain.

Then a young guy in casual clothes walked through the ER, glanced in my direction, walked over, and asked the nurse, "What's wrong with this guy?" They had a few words, and he said, "Let me take a look."

He checked the monitor, the chart, and asked me my symptoms. He then told me I was having a heart attack. "I think we can save some heart muscle. I'm going to administer a clot busting drug[1]." I had no idea what he meant. I later learned that he most probably saved my life, and saved enough of my heart muscle to salvage the rest of my life.

---

[1] I later learned he administered streptokinase, a clot-busting drug. If administered soon enough after a heart attack, this was the best approach to potentially saving additional heart muscle from damage (in 1987).

Of course, I still had the intense pain in my back, and my head still felt like it was going to explode. They administered more morphine (they had been giving me shots of morphine from the time I arrived) and, at some point, the pain started to subside. I had no idea if the pain subsided as a result of the morphine, the clot busting drugs, or that the heart attack was ending. All I knew was the pain was decreasing.

The young doctor stayed with me all day, and into the night; he was back every half-hour or so checking on me. As the day went on, I found out he was a cardiologist, it was his day off, and he just happened to be passing through the ER at the same time the crew was working on me — had Dr. Jacob Levin not passed through the ER that day, and cared enough to ask about a patient in distress, I may not be here today.

As the hours wore on, I felt better and better. Maybe it was because they kept giving me morphine—so not only was the pain gone, but I was enveloped in a blanket of relaxation, and a sense of well-being.

Late in the evening, perhaps 1 or 2 a.m., Dr. Levin, still checking on me (is this the way cardiologists spend their day off?), looks at me and says, "Do you have any questions?" I, at this point feeling pretty cocky, said to him, flippantly, "Well Doc, will I live?" He looked me straight in the eye, said something that I have never forgotten, something that changed my life, forever—"We will see."

We will see? WE WILL SEE??!! It was like he hit me right between the eyes! Have you ever been told that you might not live? Have you ever been in a situation where you realized you might not survive?

Look, I was sitting in a hospital bed, surrounded by medical professionals, a cardiologist by my side—he was young, up to date on all the latest medical advances, he had the latest technology at his disposal. The thought that I might not live really, truly hadn't crossed my mind. I was in the hospital, in the hands of a great doctor; it never occurred to me that I would not be saved—not only saved but completely cured, and hopefully in an hour or two so I could go about my business.

Had I ever faced death before? Yes, actually I had a couple near death experiences—the most dramatic being an incident that occurred when I was laying under my car, and it rolled off the bumper Jack, crashing down onto a jack stand. As it hit the jack stand, I rolled out from under the car, a split second before the jack stand collapsed and the car crashed to the ground. My chest would have been crushed, and I surely would have died. Though the incident left me seriously shaken, once it was over, it was over.

Now I was faced with the thought that my life might end, NOW. Absent a bizarre accident like a car falling on me, the thought that I might die, now, had never before crossed my mind. Of course I had thought about dying—*some*day! Not *to*day. Not *NOW*.

His proclamation had a dramatic effect on me, and it has never left me in these 26 years since the words came out of his mouth. It was a realization of my mortality. And I mean a real, actual, tangible realization. Since he told me "We will see," I have never forgotten that the day and time of my demise could be upon me, at *any* time. The effect this has had on my life has been profound.

I could die. Today, tomorrow, anytime.

The Long Morning After

I would say, "When I woke up the next morning", but I never really slept. I just drifted in a morphine induced state half-asleep.

Eventually they rolled me, not to a room, but to the CCU (Cardiac Care Unit). The CCU cares for patients immediately following heart attacks and heart surgeries, and provides immediate care should anything be out of the norm. There is much more staff than for a regular room or ward, and all are trained to deal with cardiac care. Each patient is connected to a monitor, and each bed has a small private area draped with curtains, so there is no getting away from the sound of heart monitors, alarms and nurses bustling about.

I was still on a heart monitor from the ER, so there was a bundle of wires running from me to the monitor next to the bed. I was also on intravenous fluids, so there was an IV running into a vein on the back of my hand. And my index finger was attached to a pulse/oxygen monitor.

They were slowly lessening the amount of morphine. But something they did not lessen was the nitroglycerin; it was applied as a paste, directly to the skin—just smeared on, and loosely covered by a piece of gauze—and it's absorbed right through the skin. The way nitroglycerin works, and the reason they use it in these situations, is that it "dilates" (opens up, makes wider) the arteries, thereby reducing the possibility of blockage. However, nitro isn't specific to the heart; it dilates the arteries everywhere in the body. What this means is, along with dilating the heart arteries, it also dilates the arteries in the brain; resulting in a splitting headache, a genuine pounding headache. One that doesn't subside. One that continues as long as the nitro is used. Which can be a long time. Hours, days, months, years.

After perhaps three or four days, they decided I was stable enough for further testing. In 1987 angiograms were in their infancy as a routine test; and none of the hospitals in my immediate area were equipped to do it. They arranged to transport me to a medical center in the greater Philadelphia area. An indication of the severity of my condition was the protocol surrounding the transport. Still connected to heart monitor and intravenous, I was loaded into the back of an ambulance, and sent to the hospital, some two hours away, a nurse by my side every step of the way.

An "angiogram" reveals whether there are any blockages, or narrowing, in the arteries in the heart. This is done by feeding a catheter (a long tube) through the artery in the inner thigh, up to the heart, and releasing dye in the various arteries of the heart. This dye is observed in real time on a monitor as it disburses through the artery. If there is any narrowing in the artery, it is obvious.

The patient is awake throughout, as the patient needs to cooperate and breathe, or hold their breath at the appropriate times. It is done in a Catheterization Lab, with a team of about four people, led by the doctor who actually performs the procedure. To reduce stress on the heart, the Cath Lab is kept very cool. So, in addition to being extremely nervous about the procedure, having the hair in my pubic area shaved, laying on a table naked surrounded by people I did not know, I was also freezing and shivering. Great.

They did inject me with something intravenously to help me "relax". So, once again in a drug induced stupor, I just sort of drifted through the procedure and went with the flow.

The end result—they told me there are three main arteries of the heart, and all three had blockages, one at 40 percent, one at 70 percent, and at 20 percent. This didn't sound so wonderful to me.

The day after the procedure they shipped me back to the original hospital, once again in an ambulance with a nurse. I remained in the hospital another couple weeks, while they observed me, tested me (stress test) and determined a course of treatment.

During that time, I had a series of roommates, all with cardiac problems. They were all older than me, from their late 40s to their early 60s. And they all looked pretty terrible—unhealthy, in pain. One of the roommates was a guy who had had open heart surgery, bypass; he had apparently decided that once having bypass he could eat whatever he wanted and it wouldn't be a problem. Problem was, now he clogged the bypasses. Another was a man in his late 40s, who told me this was his eighth or ninth visit to the hospital with heart problems. Is this what I had to look forward to?

Living in a hospital, receiving medical care, for any period of time has an unreal aspect to it. It's as though you've been removed from the "real world" and are living in a little world unto itself. One of the bright spots of my hospital stay was when, coincidentally, a local man about the same age as my father, who had once employed me to work part-time in his auto glass business, became my roommate. Jimmy was at least 25 years older than me, and had been admitted as he had plaque buildup in his carotid arteries.

Following the surgery, he was recovering, and just waiting for his stress test to go home. Unlike all the other roommates I had, Jimmy was in good physical shape, had a healthy and vital look about him, and had a real desire to live—he wanted out, he wanted to be home, he wanted to be going about his life. Jimmy was a good influence on me; he got me thinking about the right thing—going on with my life—getting out of the hospital. Seeing him also made me realize that I didn't necessarily have to be an unhealthy specimen, in and out of the hospital all the time, like my prior roommates.

Eventually the doctor decided that, based on my blockages, they would treat me "medically", meaning I would be given medications to treat the condition. This seemed strange to me, a lay person—the blockages certainly sounded extensive, and though I was relieved that I would not be facing open heart surgery, I was simultaneously concerned that perhaps enough wasn't being done.

I'll Never Live to See 50

During that month in the hospital I developed an appreciation for the uniqueness of my situation . . . meaning my relative youth.

When I was taken to the hospital, and in the immediate weeks following, all my focus was on the present. How I felt at that particular time, what the medical professionals were doing to me. I initially was too occupied with survival, strength and pain to give any thought to the meaning of all this. I really didn't have the time, or the inclination, to consider my situation in any light but that of the moment.

However, the longer I stayed in the hospital, the more aware I became of the uniqueness of my situation. A series of roommates all older, some considerably older, than myself. The quizzical looks from nurses when they learned my age. No other patients my age anywhere in this world of cardiac care. Finally I asked one of the nurses if it was unusual to see someone my age in this situation.

She told me that occasionally they saw young people with heart attacks, but almost always it was drug related. Specifically, she told me it was related to cocaine; apparently, misuse of cocaine can cause something known as a "cocaine heart attack", which is a heart attack brought on by a combination of the quickening of the pulse, and narrowing of the arteries, two effects of cocaine use. She told me that it was really unusual to see anyone my age, or younger, with a heart attack from "natural" causes.

And though I was a drug abuser some 20 years earlier, that had not been the case for nearly two decades. They had all my blood work, and the doctors and nurses all knew my heart attack was not drug-induced. I was one of the rare youthful victims of early heart disease, and the caregivers were all especially considerate to me.

As I said, my roommates were all older than me, and had heart attacks, like me. But the thing I did not have in common with them was that their initial heart attacks all took place much later in life than mine. In fact, most of them did not have a problem with their heart until they were at least 20 years older than me. And, it seems that once they started with heart disease, it progressed. Which is why some of them were back in the hospital for the second, third, fourth, or fifth time. (At the time, I did not realize there may have been other heart attack survivors who were doing well, and thriving. They were not the people I was sharing hospital rooms with.)

All I could think was—here I am, at 37, starting down the same road as these folks. And what do I have to look forward to? Well, apparently, a life filled with medications, some of which were very uncomfortable (the ongoing, head exploding, nitroglycerin, which was applied round-the-clock), a bland menu that you wouldn't want to feed your dog, some kind of an exercise program, and a future filled with heart attacks and hospital stays. Oh joy.

And of course, I would be just like these other people, only I was beginning the journey 20 years earlier than most. And, it was pretty obvious to me, that none of these people were going to be around for the long term—they obviously had this ongoing battle with heart disease. Seemed to me like they were all going to die. Same for me? Only 20 years earlier?

So as I looked into the future, in my mind, I could never see myself reaching 50 years old. It seemed like a very long way away. I was worried I would have another heart attack and that I would not survive—after all, a trained cardiologist couldn't tell me if I was going to make it through the first heart attack. I had no reason to believe that my future was anything other than increasing heart problems, and declining health.

After all, isn't life just an ongoing battle against death? And when we are younger our bodies are so strong, and so regenerative, that we don't even realize. But as we age we realize we are fighting, with ever-increasing intensity, to maintain our health. We all know from dealing with older members of our families that once health starts to decline, it can turn into a futile battle, with snowballing medical problems and medical complexities. Ending in only one place.

So . . . my 50th birthday . . . it seemed a million miles away. And the truth is, I absolutely believed, and I absolutely accepted, that I would never live to see 50. This was an internal truth that stayed with me, and colored my thinking and my actions, for many years. I just didn't, and don't, have the luxury to procrastinate . . . not on anything of importance.

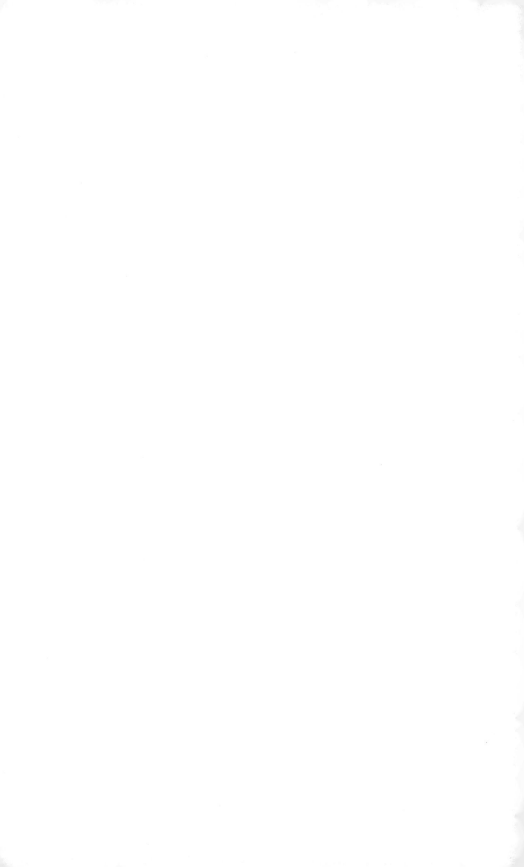

How Could This Happen? Why Me?

How could this happen at age 37? Being 6'1" tall and weighing 170 pounds? Clearly, I was too young, too thin, and in too good condition to have a heart attack. I had never heard of anyone in my family having a heart attack, young. Matter-of-fact, I had never heard of anyone in my family having a heart attack at all.

I learned there were several major risk factors:
- ♥ Heredity. We don't get to pick our parents. We inherit our genes, and there's nothing we can do about it.
- ♥ What you eat. It has a direct effect on the levels of LDL ("bad cholesterol") in your blood.
- ♥ Weight. Too much is no good, and raises the risk of heart attack.
- ♥ Exercise, or the lack thereof. Exercise has many benefits, but one of them is that it increases HDL (the "good cholesterol").
- ♥ Smoking. This has a devastating effect on health, and on heart health.
- ♥ Stress. Uncontrolled stress or anger can be bad, very bad.

And how did these factors apply to me?

Heredity. Well, there's nothing I could do about my genes. What I knew about my family history really didn't indicate there was any early onset of heart disease. Sure, there were older folks in my family who eventually had congestive heart failure; but this is when they were in their advanced years and in failing health. So not having a history of early-onset heart disease left me wondering how this could happen.[2]

---

[2] Decades later I learned that my father's father died at 45. They say it was a heart attack, though there was no autopsy.

What I ate consisted of whatever tasted best, lots of sugar and fat. I gave no regard to nutritional value, only that it satisfied my appetite and tasted good. The trouble with this approach was, when they took me into the hospital on the day of my heart attack, my cholesterol was over 300! Prior, I had never had my cholesterol checked—why should I? I was young and in good health! So on the first risk factor that was under my control, I failed miserably; my cholesterol was three times the desired level!

Weight. Here my genes helped me, because there was certainly nothing I was doing to control my weight. My eating was out of control. I was able to stuff myself with all those things that caused others to break out in fat, and that dentists said make your teeth fall out. And yet I was thin, and had teeth.

Exercise. Yes, I did exercise on and off over the years, but it was all strength training aimed at certain muscles or muscle groups. None of it was focused on my cardiovascular system. I heard of "aerobic exercise", but I thought it was for women who wanted to lose weight, as the only aerobic exercise I ever heard of was "aerobic exercise classes", which were attended by women. I don't think I ever rode my bike, jogged or swam so long and hard that my heart was really pumping; I didn't think I needed that. After all, I was thin. So on another risk factor that I could've controlled, I also failed miserably.

Smoking. Of course I knew smoking was not good for my health, as does everyone who smokes. For whatever reason, I thought I could get away with it—maybe it was that I grew up in a time when many adults smoked, cigarette ads were all over the TV, Humphrey Bogart, Steve McQueen and lots of other Hollywood stars looked pretty cool smoking, and it wasn't really as unacceptable as it is today. Nonetheless, everyone who smoked knew it was bad for their health. And I had been smoking since I was about 14 or 15 years old, 20 years or so. And I smoked a lot. Two packs of cigarettes a day. So again, I failed to control this risk factor.

Stress. I was a vice president in a banking organization, and my job at that time had to do with installing and managing ATMs, finding and building new ATM sites, making sure that customers had ATM cards and were using them. There were about 30 people who reported to me . . . including a subsidiary armored car company. I had the normal insane stress that all middle managers do—personnel, budget, hours, projects. But I also had about ten people out on the streets every day armed with guns, in a business that was a historic target of armed robbers. Only unlike bank robberies, armored car robberies nearly always result in deaths. I thought I managed the stress well; in hindsight, this was not the case.

So on all the risk factors I *could* have controlled, I didn't. Had I controlled them heart attack may never have happened.

Clogged arteries can kill me. I can't control my genes, but I can control exercise, smoking, stress and what I eat.

Even knowing these things, I still had the question: Why me? There seem to be plenty of other people walking around, not exercising, not eating properly, under lots of stress, and they weren't having heart attacks.

"The Great One" — Why can't I have his life?

About this time I was sitting in a doctor's office, reading an article about the TV star, Jackie Gleason. Gleason was a big heavy man who had endeared himself to the public by portraying "Ralph Kramden", a hilarious but oftentimes pathetic "everyman" on the 1950s TV show, "The Honeymooners" (which Gleason created, wrote, directed and starred in). By the 80s Gleason had starred in movies, had his own TV variety show, and was often referred to as "The Great One", a nickname given him by Orson Welles.

Gleason had passed away recently, and the article discussed his lifestyle. He kept long hours, sometimes not sleeping at all because he was partying all night. He was morbidly obese (over 300 pounds), but he happily maintained a diet of excess, heavily laden with juicy steaks, multiple times a day—his obit in the New York Times mentions he could eat 5 lobsters at one sitting! He smoked—but he smoked to the same excess as everything else, 5 packs a day. 5 packs a day! He drank excessively—the better term would be "legendarily", because again, he was beyond excess, downing bottles of fine Scotch daily.

He lived a life of little sleep, and grossly excess eating, drinking, smoking and partying, and yet he lived into his 70s. How is it he could get away with this lifestyle, and yet I, at age 37, thin and relatively fit looking, was having a heart attack? It just wasn't fair.

What it took me a really long time to accept was, life really isn't fair. And, there's nothing you can do about it. It seems there are always people who can get away with doing things that you can't. I slowly realized I must accept that this is the hand I was dealt, and move on; denial of reality could only lead to a life of discontent.

Life is not always fair.

"This Is What You Need To Change"

When I was finally released from the hospital, I was ecstatic, I was going home. Being in the hospital for a nearly month was almost like being on another planet. I saw my wife on a regular basis, but had only seen the kids a few times during the entire month. I had absolutely no contact with work; very unusual as I did hold a responsible position, with a number of subordinates, and was of course concerned about both my position and the condition of the business. And, I was anxious to go for a ride on my motorcycle. I was really ready to go home.

That morning, my nurse went over the instructions about what I was supposed to do:

1. Stop smoking. Even though I had smoked, heavily, for 20 years this didn't seem like a problem. I had spent the last month in wards, floors, and rooms equipped with oxygen, where smoking was not permitted. So it had already been 30 days without a cigarette.

2. Go to "cardiac rehab". Well, I didn't know what this was, but how bad could it be?

3. Exercise my cardiovascular system, regularly. Now, at the time, I was 6'1", 170 pounds, so I was not the kind of person that needed to exercise to keep my weight under control. I did do a little bit of strength training, but that was all focused on forearm and wrist strength, and shoulder, neck and back strength for riding motorcycles. And I did it when I wanted; I was certainly not on a rigid schedule.

4. Go for a weekly blood test. I was apparently on some kind of blood thinner, and there was a risk of internal bleeding if the dosage was incorrect. Therefore, every week they

would draw blood and adjust the dosage if necessary. (I didn't know it at the time, but being on the blood thinner would have an impact on other aspects of my life.)

5. Change what I eat. Well, I didn't think this would be a big deal until they told me what they wanted me to do!!
   - ♥ Low sodium
   - ♥ Low fat
   - ♥ Low cholesterol
   - ♥ Low sugar
   - ♥ No caffeine

OMG! Low-fat? Low-sodium? Low sugar? No coffee? Were these people kidding? From the time I left my parents' home, some 20 years prior, I had survived on a menu of all the things I loved. Things like Frosted Flakes, Fruit Loops and Pop Tarts for breakfast, Italian salami sandwiches for lunch, steak for dinner. Anything that was grown by farmers was simply not on my plate.

And let me tell you, I really loved what I ate. I always had a "fast metabolism", so I never had a problem with weight. Sitting in bed at night, reading a book, and eating a half a box of graham crackers and milk was the norm — unless I was eating Girl Scout thin mints, or Ring Dings or Twinkies.

And these people are telling me low sugar, low-fat, low cholesterol, low-sodium? Well, this eliminated *everything* that I ate at the time!

Big Bill Tilden says . . .

Bill Tilden may have been the greatest tennis player who ever lived. You never heard of Tilden, and yet I am asserting he is one of the greats?

Tilden was the world's No. 1 player for seven years, and dominated the world of international tennis in the 1920s. In 1950, when the Associated Press named "The Greatest Athletes of the Half Century", people like Babe Ruth and Jim Thorpe, Bill Tilden was named the greatest tennis player by a margin greater than any other athlete in any sport. (It should also be mentioned that at the close of the 20th century, ESPN named Tilden one of the Top 100 American Athletes of the century; in fact, they ranked him higher than any other male tennis player.)

However, except for the sports writers and statisticians, Tilden quietly slipped into obscurity. I only heard of him because I followed tennis, and when I was much younger heard a sports commentator refer to him as the greatest who had ever played the game. Somehow, I came across his long-out-of-print book, "How To Play Better Tennis"; I scarfed it up. It is a great book for anyone who wants to play better tennis, and it helped me tremendously with the game.

One of Tilden's lessons that stuck with me was on strategy:

Never change a winning game.

Always change a losing game.

The first seems obvious. You would think that anyone would know enough to follow that rule, but for some perverse reason it seems to work the other way with some players. A player will build up a winning lead by staying back and pounding his opponent. Then suddenly, for no understandable reason, he begins to rush the net, starts losing points, and ends by being defeated.

Conversely, it is equally stupid to insist upon playing to the end a type of game that is losing badly. If you do, you are certain to lose. You may lose anyway, but you might better try to win with something else. Try out something new, if what you have previously been trying has failed.

I have applied Tilden's axiom to many aspects of both my personal life and professional life. It is so simple, and has made such a huge difference. Regarding heart disease, I never realized I was playing a losing game—but once I did I also realized that if I didn't change, I was going to lose, in a really big way.

Never change a winning game.
Always change a losing game.

part two
recovery

First Steps

When I was finally released from the hospital after nearly a month, I was told to go for weekly blood tests, not smoke, eat correctly, start a program of cardiac rehabilitation, stay calm, and see the doctor in two weeks. Truth is, I felt okay, although physically weak, and mentally shaken.

My first meeting with the cardiologist brought a big surprise. In addition to all the things I was supposed to avoid, he added motorcycles to the list. He told me that with the blood thinner in my system, if I was to go down and get a brush burn, it is unlikely there would be any way to stop the bleeding—so the way he saw it, riding a motorcycle while taking a blood thinner presented an enormous risk . . . of bleeding to death.

Hmmm, the most relaxing thing I did, the thing that let me clear my head of all the conflicts and stresses, was cruising down the road on my bike. Can't smoke, can't eat, can't ride—great, it's getting shittier by the minute. So I walked in there feeling okay, and I walked out feeling terrible, like the things I loved in life were slipping further and further away.

A few days later, I visited my primary care physician, a doctor I had known for a long time and trusted. This visit also brought a big surprise. After examining me and looking over the records, he asked me if I knew how long my company disability would cover me. I had excellent benefits—and I knew they would pay me full salary for up to six months. He told me I was going to be out of work for the entire six months.

Well, I really didn't feel so sick that I thought I needed six months to recover. As a matter of fact, I didn't feel terribly sick at all. I felt more tired, shaken, and scared than I felt sick—and I told him that. He advised me that following a medical event as dramatic as a myocardial infarction, I should give myself every opportunity to recover and rehabilitate, physically, mentally, and emotionally. So I walked out of there wondering what I was going to spend the next five months doing; from the time I started kindergarten I had never had 5 months off!

Once I got my head around the idea of extended absence from work, I realized I could focus on my cardiac rehab, and on understanding my new eating requirements (which I still hated). I also realized that, as I regained my strength, I'd be able to do some small projects on my Harley, even though I couldn't ride it (or could I?); there was nothing stopping me from working on it in the garage, and I also found that extremely relaxing.

The next week I began cardiac rehab. This was another of those interesting experiences, where I looked around the room and discovered all the other patients were old enough to be my father, or maybe my grandfather. There was no one my age, or anywhere close to it. The idea of cardiac rehab is, first, to get used to the idea of exercising; second, to help (safely and progressively) to build the capacity to exercise—which should ultimately build the confidence to use the heart, to exercise, without undue fear or risk.

At the rehab facility, you are connected to a pulse monitor, which tracks your heart rate as you exercise. Typically the exercise is done on a treadmill, where you begin to walk at a modest pace and the pace slowly picks up until you hit the target heart rate. And you need to stay at the target heart rate for a certain period of time.

Occasionally, instead of directing me to the treadmill the therapist used a different machine. One day when my back was sore, and I didn't think I could walk for the required amount of time, they sat me at a table in front of a device that looked like a pair of bicycle pedals. But these pedals were operated with the hands and arms, cranking them around in circles against adjustable resistance—and the purpose was the same, to achieve the target heart rate for a specified period of time. And there are other machines—bikes, rowing machines, ellipticals, etc.

Once I figured out that the idea was to bring the heart to an increased rate, for a specified period of time, I started to ask questions about how the target heart rate was determined, and how the length of time was determined. Once I had the answers, I became a "cardiac rehab dropout"—after all, did I really need to travel a half hour and hang out with a bunch of old men to get my heart rate up? There was simply no reason I could not supervise my own rehab.

There were two activities that could bring up my heart rate that I actually enjoyed—bicycling and walking. Lucky for me, the heart attack happened in the summer, so I had August, September and October to enjoy the outdoors before winter. And, also lucky for me, a half block from our home was a rails-to-trails conversion— yep, a "bicycle path" that ran for miles through four adjacent towns.

So I started bicycling every day, for about an hour. And this was an hour that I never believed I had in my day before, I was simply "too busy". Since I wasn't working, I had no excuse—there was no reason that I couldn't, or shouldn't, exercise for an hour every day. And, I really like bicycling. The unexpected result was, months later after I had returned to work and to my normal life, I had developed the habit and understood the necessity for daily exercise. To this very day, 26 years later, I try to exercise every day (the reality is, now, I average about five days a week).

I was exercising every day, I was going to occasional doctor appointments, and I was having a weekly blood test to determine if my blood was being thinned enough, but not too much. If the dosage of blood thinner is too high there is a risk of internal bleeding, so as long as the patient is on a blood thinner there are regular tests.

Being on the blood thinner also meant I shouldn't ride my motorcycle, because of the risk of falling, and bleeding uncontrollably. The more I thought about it, the more I realized that if I could reduce the risk, I should be able to ride the motorcycle.

I decided there were two ways to lower the risk. The first, protective gear—this was not a problem, as I already had a jacket, gloves, boots and chaps. This however did not bring the risk factor down where I wanted—because the biggest risk to motorcyclists is not merely falling over, the biggest risk to motorcyclists is cars. I needed the roads to myself, with no cars on them.

I thought about middle of the night rides, but these carry the risk of drunks leaving bars at 2 a.m. after "last call". So what I decided was 5:30 a.m. was going to be "ride time"—and if I went out that early I could be back by 7:30, before any heavy traffic. I also decided that the risk increased by how often I rode—so I limited the rides to twice a week. I never mentioned this to the doctor, because I didn't want him to think that I wasn't taking the situation seriously, but my psychological well-being was equally important, and somehow motorcycling filled a void in my psyche.

The dawn rides worked for the couple months until they stopped the blood thinner. And once that happened, my recovery actually became fun. Not working but collecting a full paycheck, the only real responsibility was my daily exercise, and this was a responsibility to me, not others. And, I could ride again.

The remainder of my time off was very pleasant. Daily exercise—and sometimes this was riding my bicycle on the path near home, at other times I would load the bicycle onto the car and take it to the boardwalk in Atlantic City. (I have always loved bicycling on the boardwalk, with the thumpity-thump of the tires over the boards, the sound of the surf, and the feel of the salt air.) Reflecting—sometimes I would find myself sitting on a bench, in the sun, just enjoying being alive. I had never really considered how amazing it was to be alive before and had never really appreciated it—now, I enjoyed real happiness sitting quietly on a bench in the sun.

Motorcycling—I was a member of the local ABATE chapter. ABATE is the American Bikers Aimed to Educate, and the purpose was to defend motorcyclists from discriminatory legislation and practices, but in reality it was a social group. Suddenly I had time to attend the meetings and show up at the events. I loved motorcycling, and really liked the members, so I now had the opportunity to enjoy motorcycling in a different way.

The only downside was, I was starting to enjoy myself so much that I wasn't really anxious to go back to work. Full pay and leisure time, what could be better? But the reality was, this was a recovery period, not an escape.

And what came out of the extended recovery period were several things of great value. Exercise became a daily habit, which has stuck with me. My commitment to a very healthy way of eating crystallized, and that also has stuck with me through the years. My ability to appreciate the wonder of life, and enjoy the simple things—the sunlight, the laughter of my son and daughter—developed in a way that it never had before. The understanding that some things truly are "life and death" matters—and other things, like spats with relatives, "emergencies" at work, broken plumbing, are really not, and are not worth getting upset over (when you have looked death in the eye, it puts everything else in perspective).

RELAX.
Most upsetting things are really not "life and death", and not worth getting stressed.

My primary care doctor was right, taking six months to recover went a long way at healing me physically and emotionally. It let me develop the attitudes and habits I needed to manage my health in a different way for the rest of my life. I realize how fortunate I was to have such excellent benefits, and also realize everyone does not. But the advice to take as much time as possible and devote it to a slow steady recovery was one of the best pieces of advice I ever received. So I pass it on to you—take as much time as you possibly can, there is nothing more important than your recovery.

Being away from work that long was also interesting, not just in terms of the reduced stress from being out of the day-to-day, but being away from the normal daily social interactions. Interestingly, some of my colleagues went out of their way to stay in touch, or even help . . . and others acted like I had the plague.

"Mr. Atlantic City"

A few years prior my Dad passed on, losing a four year battle to cancer. I watched him slowly slip away, turning from an energetic humorous 180-pound extrovert, eventually to a 95-pound invalid. But the change was slow, very slow. As time went on there were less and less "good days" when he could do what he liked, interspersed with more and more bad days of pain and low energy . . . always getting weaker, frailer, sicker, closer to the inevitable.

Well, Dad had an interesting life, having served in the Marine Corps in WWII, serving as a councilman and commissioner in our town, and serving as the chairman of the Committee To Legalize Gambling in New Jersey. This was the public face; the private face was . . . he was a compulsive gambler, who spent the majority of his spare time in card games in smoke filled rooms. So, let's say between the Marines, politics, and gambling, he had some "interesting" friends.

One of his friends was "Mr. Atlantic City", Paul "Skinny" D'Amato, the owner of The 500 Club, and undisputed king of the entertainment world in Atlantic City. Skinny discovered Dean Martin and Jerry Lewis. He was Frank Sinatra's best friend. He was well known in Hollywood. Any major entertainer who wanted to play Atlantic City called him. Strikingly handsome, gorgeous wife, thousand dollar shoes, beautiful home. Skinny lived the life of a celebrity, rubbing elbows with the rich and famous.

He was also, reputedly, tied to "the mob"; I don't really know the truth of that, but I do know that Skinny, like Dad, was a gambler. I also know that somehow their round-the-clock card games, whether they were in the back room at the 500 Club, Skinny's home, or our home (where there was a dedicated "card room" with roulette wheel, felt covered card table, craps table, bar) were never noticed by the authorities. And this is what they did— gamble.

When others were devoting time to their families, their hobbies, their interests, my Dad, Skinny, their buddies, and the "fish" they could reel in, were locked in smoke-filled rooms. My Dad, and I'm sure Skinny, had this perverse idea that if the game was at their house, they were spending time with their family—hey Dad!, hey, Skinny!, if you're locked up in the card room for 12 hours that doesn't count! (Sorry, but I was too young or polite to say it when I was a kid.)

So while others saw Skinny as a glamorous impresario surrounded by stars and starlets, I knew Skinny as just one more of my Dad's buddies who was sequestered in the card room, ever present cigarette hanging from his lip. I've heard it said that Skinny was a man of few words—I knew Skinny for 25 years, from the time I was 10 until his passing. In those 25 years I don't recall Skinny ever saying anything to me—he may have grunted a greeting in passing. Perhaps he was too busy (for 25 years?), maybe he didn't like kids, or maybe he didn't have time for the social graces beyond those necessary for his business.

But my overall impression of him was, he was unfriendly, reeked of the smell of gambling halls (cigarettes and booze), dressed in expensive gangster clothes that normal people didn't wear, and always had a general look of being up to something. And he was part of that other, negative world of Dads'. I didn't like him.

In 1978 my Dad started his four year battle with cancer. Between his decades long involvement in politics and network of gambling contacts he had a small army of "friends". People who came to our home for political cocktail parties, people who went on trips with my parents, people who we were told to address as "Aunt" or "Uncle". Initially, all these people called, and came, to show support for Dad.

But time dragged on—days became weeks became months became years. And Dad got weaker, and thinner, as time passed. By year three it was bad; occasionally he would have a "good day"—he would don his Stetson, put on silk slacks and a sport coat (which all now looked two sizes too large), and go to one of the casinos. One of the casinos that only existed due to his efforts to legalize gambling!

And as time passed, and he didn't recover, the parade of "friends" showing support thinned. First went the political cronies, then went the gamblers. It's really tough to watch someone wither away, and if you're not truly a friend. . . . Eventually there were only a few, and they were mostly family.

I had taken to stopping to visit Dad most days on the way home from work, about 6 p.m. But this particular day I left work early, maybe 3. When I entered the house, it seemed empty, so I walked through, and spotted Dad sitting under a tree in the back corner of the yard, talking . . . with Skinny. And off in the other corner was the big guy who seemed to always be with Skinny, Poochie (or Pucci?—I was never quite sure); I think he was Skinny's bodyguard. I didn't want to intrude, so I just moseyed on.

The next day I mentioned it to Dad, and he told me that Skinny walked over to see him every afternoon. Skinny only lived about four blocks away, but he was 74 years old at the time, and also didn't look too great. And I realized then that my dislike had been unjustified; here, near the end, was one of the true friends. A man so loyal that he could tolerate the pain of seeing a friend fade away, of seeing a friend slowly losing his vitality and his essence. My opinion of Skinny changed to admiration and respect.

During the six months I was recovering I heard from good friends—but mysteriously some who I thought were good friends were just plain absent. Perhaps their lives were too busy to pay a visit to a sick friend, perhaps they were uncomfortable dealing with illness—I don't know. But I do know that times of trouble, times of illness, will separate the true friends from the others—and that may be the source of both pleasant surprise and unexpected disappointment.

Slow Adjustments

Shouldn't be so hard (ha-ha)—they said stop smoking, exercise, and eat healthful foods. Outside of that, I needed to take my pills and observe certain precautions that apply to every heart patient.

So let's start with the first one—stop smoking. I had spent nearly a month in intensive care and cardiac units; these places all had oxygen, so no smoking was permitted. Though I had been a heavy smoker (two packs a day) I had not had a cigarette in a month, so I knew, deep down, I had physically "kicked the habit". Regardless, I still longed for a cigarette.

Certain times of day, and certain activities, seemed to trigger the need/yearning/addiction, and at those times it was overwhelming. Also, when I was near someone who was smoking the cigarette smoke was unbearable—and I don't mean in a bad way, the cigarette smelled so good it was all I could think about. But I knew, I knew, I had physically kicked the habit . . . so why was it so hard?

It was, of course, the psychological addiction. Even though my body no longer craved the nicotine, my mind kept insisting I should smoke.

So first I attempted "substitutions". Something healthy, sunflower seeds or the like. I went looking for sunflower seeds, pumpkin seeds, or anything like that that I could chew on whenever I craved a cigarette. I tried this for several weeks, it was an abject failure—when your body is craving a stimulant, the last thing it wants is to be chewing is a totally nondescript, tasteless object. (This was before research revealed the heart-healthy nature of some of my favorite nuts.)

Then I decided that the real problem with cigarettes was inhaling the nicotine into my lungs, hence into my system. So maybe what I could do is smoke, but not inhale—which led me to the idea of pipe smoking.

From the time I was a youngster, I always loved the smell of those aromatic pipe tobaccos—not all pipe tobaccos, just the aromatic ones. I researched pipes, and decided to go with a purely American choice, a corncob. I went to the tobacco store in my town, where they had shelves full of tobacco, in glass jars, with names like "Blue Rain", "Amaretto", "Irish Oak", "Red Toro" and "Guilty Pleasure". The proprietor helped me pick out two or three of the aromatic blends to try.

Well, talk about a shock! Those aromatic tobaccos smell great, but the taste is nothing like the smell. The taste of pipe tobacco is strong, and has a "bite". I spent the next several months trying to try to find one that had a taste that wasn't completely disgusting, and had no bite. To actually smoke a pipe is also very different than you would imagine; it's not like a cigarette or a cigar, which gets lit and smoked. No, the smoker must pack the pipe bowl with tobacco, tamp it down, light it—take a few puffs, go about your business for a few seconds, come back and try to take another puff—that's when you discover it has gone out. So you re-light the pipe, tamp it, puff it—over and over and over.

What I actually learned from pipe smoking was: First, no matter how good the tobacco smells when someone else is smoking it, it's not going to taste good; in fact, it's harsh, bitter and nasty. Additionally, though it likely doesn't contribute to heart disease, it certainly does contribute to mouth and throat cancer. And last, the amount of time and effort you must devote to smoking a pipe is completely disproportionate to any benefit.

My ultimate solution for smoking was very straightforward. I told myself that this was just like the people who attend AA, and know that they just should not take the next drink; not start thinking about that they could never have a drink for the rest of their life, just focus on "Don't take the next drink". My approach, and it has been successful for 26 years, has been to not smoke the next cigarette. That's it—just don't smoke the *next* cigarette.

Just don't smoke the *next* cigarette.

It did, honestly, take me years to get over the idea that I wanted a cigarette. I kept a pack in the glove compartment of the car, just in case I had another heart attack, was rushed to the hospital dying, and needed to have that "last cigarette". Even though I never smoked another cigarette, I kept that pack in the glove compartment for about five years—at some point, the craving stopped, and I threw away the very stale pack of cigarettes.

Then there's exercise, something I hated almost as much as I loved cigarettes. I don't know about you, but I was one of the kids that hated gym in school. There were a few reasons—first, I wasn't very good at athletics. Second, they made you do calisthenics and exercises, and I was lazy and didn't like to get sweaty. Third, when I did the exercises I realized I wasn't one of the strong kids—in fact I was one of the weak kids who got tired easily and whose muscles started to hurt. Now apparently there was no choice. Exercise or die.

It wasn't like I had an extra hour or two in my day. I had a job, family, interests, responsibilities . . . these things took up the whole day. In fact, they took up more than the whole day—it seemed like there was never a day when I went to bed that there were not things yet undone. So when was I going to find the time to exercise?

There were physical activities that I liked. Primarily bicycling and walking. But anything that seemed like formal, structured exercise really turned me off. And to complicate things, I had several back operations when I was in my 20s, which prevented me from doing certain things, including jogging, running, tennis, golf, skiing. My quest to find the right exercise program was not as challenging as stopping smoking. I knew from the beginning what it was going to be—walking and bicycling. The real problem was finding the time and place, daily.

My solution for this was also very straightforward. I just told myself, and everyone around me, that I needed to exercise every day—and it didn't matter whether I was home on a regular day, away on a business trip, or even on a motorcycle trip with friends. When at home, I had a certain schedule and routine for when I would exercise. When on business or pleasure trips I would start each day with a brisk walk; sometimes I was in a beautiful locale where I could walk outside and enjoy the scenery, but if not I tried to be in a hotel or motel that had exercise facilities and a treadmill.

As much as I hate to admit it, I learned that exercise actually made me feel better. And I don't mean just over the long term in helping maintain my health, I mean the short term—after I exercise I am more alert, more awake, and my day goes better than if I had not exercised. (Don't get me wrong, I still hate exercise.)

Somehow or other, I have managed to fit exercise into most days. I try to walk for about 40 minutes, so it takes about an hour out of my day. Though I haven't kept historic track of my exercise sessions I would say over the past 26 years I have exercised at least four or five days a week.

Do I like it? No. Do I do it? Yes.

Jack LaLanne, the fitness guru, died in 2011 at 97 years old. I saw him on TV over the years promoting fitness, and in later years promoting a "juicer" he manufactured. LaLanne owned health clubs, had a TV show, competed in bodybuilding (beating even the young Arnold Schwarzenegger at one time!), was always guest starring on the morning TV shows. I remember watching him when he was in his 70s, swimming, with a rope tied from him to a string of 70 (yes, 70) rowboats each holding a passenger, as he towed these boats for a mile in front of the Queen Mary in Long Beach, California. An amazing man. A fit man. A man with energy we all wish we could have.

I saw him interviewed one morning. He must have been in his eighties, but still healthy, vital, engaging. The interviewer asked if he still worked out. I'll never forget what he said; it was something like, "I work out for two hours every morning, seven days a week, even when I'm traveling—and I hate every minute of it!"

I still hate exercise, but I admit that it makes me feel better. And it helps keep me alive.

Impact on Family and Friends

There are three distinct groups here—friends and colleagues, blood relatives, and immediate family—and the impact on them ranges from casual to intense.

My colleagues and friends . . . do not share my genetics. They did, however, share my work environment, and we all "enjoyed" the same daily stresses. Some of them were concerned that if this could happen to someone as young and seemingly healthy as me, it could happen to them.

My longtime friend and respected colleague, Colleen, said something I've never forgotten: "Stu, the only difference between you and everyone else is that you know what's going on, and the rest of us don't." Colleen is the same age as me, and though women in their late 30s don't generally suffer heart attacks, she saw her doctor and insisted on a fasting lipid profile to check her cholesterol. Though many of my friends and colleagues expressed real concern that they could experience what I did, she was one of the few that actually followed through.

I've often wondered about the psychology of decisions like this. Some people must, absolutely must, know if there is something wrong with them—while other people prefer not to know. A few years back I saw a study that quantified the mortality rate that resulted from a conscious decision made by the person who died; it seems a huge percentage, something like 70 percent, of the people who die in the U.S. do so as a result of their own bad decisions. The number one bad decision is, apparently, deciding to not wear a seatbelt; but another bad decision that had huge implications was deciding to not get necessary medical tests. I suppose for some there's comfort in not knowing—and others like Colleen would rather know, and deal with it.

My blood relatives . . . were concerned with the obvious—we come from the same gene pool. My cholesterol at the time of the heart attack was over 300, so most of my blood relatives had their cholesterol checked. We learned that, oddly, people that share the same genetics, and even the same diet, may not have the same blood chemistry—their cholesterol results may vary drastically.

My two children were 10 and 12 years old at the time. While they did not eat the exact same food, they certainly did eat the same breakfast, and the same dinner, daily. At that age, they were both very active; this is relevant because activity and exercise affects HDL (good cholesterol). Their results could not have been more different. Our son, a laid-back 12-year-old, had great results—meaning his LDL (bad cholesterol) was very low, and his HDL was high; the exact results desired for heart health. On the other hand our daughter, an outgoing 10-year-old, had the opposite results—high LDL, low HDL. Now, I remind you, these are two children who share the same parents, lived in the same household, and ate the same food. And the results could not have been more different, so the message is, don't assume if this didn't affect your parents, or your siblings, or your cousins, that it's not going to affect you.

My immediate family . . . was, of course, most affected. Immediately, drastically, deeply, and for the long term. The immediate impact was my serious medical condition, and this was followed by living with me and all the changes in my eating, exercise and daily routine. Suddenly they were living with someone with a medical condition, with needs, with potential risks. Though none of us knew it initially, they would be dealing with long-term major changes that resulted from my realization of mortality.

My wife went from living with someone who survived on junk food and cigarettes, to living with the polar opposite. I was compulsive with my abusive habits, and was no less compulsive with my new situation. Thank goodness, she never said "I told you so", or anything like that; as a matter of fact she jumped in and did everything possible to make the transition as painless as possible. By the time I got home from the hospital there were no cookies, candy bars, ice cream, whole milk, etc., etc., anywhere in the home. Her approach was that everyone in the house would eat the same healthy foods from that time forward.

My children were probably most affected. Samantha, my daughter, was 10 years old at the time. Now, as an adult, she tells me the heart attack was significant in shaping much of her approach to life, to her "carpe diem" attitude. She says watching me deal with it taught her "Wisdom is knowing the right thing to do. Virtue is doing it." (I think this is the first time anyone ever told me I'm virtuous!) She also tells me by the time she was 18 she made a conscious decision to get to know me as well as possible, so that if anything happened and I was suddenly gone, she would know exactly how I would answer any question. Clearly my heart attack extinguished that warm fuzzy feeling we all have that our parent would always be around to provide love and support.

My son, Stephen, is a professional journalist and editor. Rather than me telling you how he was affected, I asked him to remember the impact, 26 years ago.

This is what Stephen had to say:

Kids have a tendency to be in awe of their fathers, I think, and I was no different. My dad had a deep voice, a no-nonsense attitude, and, of course, he knew every single thing in the entire world: how to fix cars and houses, who that actor was on Star Trek, what was the optimal day of the year to plant the garden, and whether I'd been poking around his record collection when he wasn't looking. So I loved and respected my father, but it was not lost on my grade-school brain that "dad" and "god" were similar-sounding words to describe the all-powerful being who you didn't want to piss off.

I was 12, a week away from finishing sixth grade, when Dad had his heart attack. I don't remember the day perfectly; I do remember I was seated at the dinner table when Mom hurried through the room, told my sister and me that Dad wasn't feeling well and she was taking him to the hospital. It was a rare and worrisome thing; we were a healthy family, all our medical visits (in my experience, at least) having been routine pediatric excursions. Mom and Dad didn't do sick—so when they were still at the hospital the next morning, it was a massive break from normal life.

Mom broke the news that day simply, with matter-of-fact concern: Dad had a heart attack, it was very serious but he was doing better today, he'd be at the hospital for some days to come and she didn't know yet how long. I don't specifically remember exactly how she phrased the words "He could have died," but I do remember being simultaneously comforted and chilled by her carefully calm "It's lucky that I'd been worried about this sort of thing and already knew what those symptoms meant."

I had utter trust in my parents as a fundamental premise of my existence; I never doubted what they told me. It was startling to learn that my father could in any way be fragile.

From my perspective as a middle-school kid, the fact that Dad's heart attack coincided with the end of our school year meant there was a sort of organic flow to the changes that came to our house: Sixth grade ended, and the new patterns of summer life started, including a father who'd also be staying home for months in an extended break from his daily grind; a new household diet that saw the prompt elimination of sugared soda, chocolate-covered graham crackers and high-cholesterol anything from our kitchen; and the disappearance of cigarette smoke from the air we breathed.

The dietary changes were an adjustment, but Mom was dedicated to showing us we could happily eat healthier versions of almost everything worth eating—with less salt, less sugar and less fat—and while I always remained happy to indulge in rich foods when the opportunity presented itself, I find that, 26 years later in adulthood, most of the basic lessons have stuck. Today I almost never drink soda; I prefer simple home recipes with raw-food ingredients to overly processed factory-food products; in the grocery store, I'm automatically inclined to reach for the healthier of any two variations of the same item. Yes, I eat too much cheese—but, overall, I'm forced to conclude that the extreme dietary shift that Dad had to endure after his heart attack meant that I internalized young how important it was to my health not to eat unthinkingly like a stereotypical gluttonous American.

Then there was the fact that Dad stopped smoking. Honestly, this might have been the most immediately profound impact on my life at the time—even more than having Dad home from work all those extra hours that summer. I'd been acclimated all my childhood to the bitter funk of cigarettes; I never liked it, but I took it for granted. Then it stopped, and I discovered two things: Our home was a lot more pleasant when it didn't smell like that, and I didn't constantly have a runny nose anymore. The latter took a little bit of time to notice, but once I did, it was like a cartoon light bulb popping up over my head: Hey, I'm not a born mucus machine! That may sound trivial, but to me it wasn't at all; I was a kid who always needed to know where the Kleenex was. (I'd been carrying it around in my pockets for years like Luke Skywalker carried his light saber; I'd tried to convince myself they were comparable accessories.) I was sorry Dad had to have a heart attack for us to discover this, and yet I was relieved to discover it.

And then there was Dad himself. It's funny how memory works; I don't remember the first time I talked to him after the heart attack, and I don't remember the moment he first came home from the hospital. What I remember most strongly is standing together in the front lawn months later, when he was beginning to think concretely about going back to work again after a summer full of bicycling and gardening, and he wanted to explain to me that he had a new understanding of time. "Right now," he said, "it's August the third, 1987, at two-thirty-three and fourteen seconds. And now it's not. And it never will be again. One of the things I've learned in the past couple months is how important it is to actually notice those moments, to step back and enjoy them for what they are, because you only get one chance."

I remembered that.

I turned 13 the next year. I don't know whether it was simply the inevitable natural rhythms of age, or whether our new awareness of Dad's mortality changed how either of us approached our father-son relationship, but in the following several years as I progressed through teenagerdom, I began to find that we consciously enjoyed each others' company in a way that had never been possible for me, at least, when as a small child I'd thought of him as the Lord Almighty. We talked more, we listened to each other more, we laughed together more. So, as a selfish, greedy son, I'll say this terrible thing: If the heart attack helped Dad and I become better friends, I'm glad it happened.

Medications

There really are two things to think about with medications — first, what are they supposed to do *for* you? And second, what else might they do *to* you? Let me answer the second question first, as it seems that everyone is always concerned about side effects.

The first unexpected thing my medications did happened about two weeks after I got out of the hospital, when I went to the local pharmacy to pick up my prescriptions; the pharmacist gave me the invoice, which almost caused a second heart attack! The medications that I had been getting for free (sort of) in the hospital were going to be $187 a month. $187 a month! In 1987 dollars! I had a medical plan and a prescription plan, but when I started to ask questions about the high cost of the medications I learned about "brand names" and patents. Seems when a great drug is still protected by patent, before it becomes "generic", it sells at a high premium — because it can be manufactured by only the patent holder, who has a monopoly on it until expiration of the patent. At that point, I became determined to outlive the patents (it never dawned on me that there would always be newer, better medications, with new patents).

Back to the real side effects: Below I've included the known reported potential side effects from one, just one, of the medications I take. I selected this medication at random, not because its side effects are any worse or any more extensive than my other medications — in fact, after doing a little more research I learned some of my other medications have much more severe side effects.

So here are the side effects of ramipril, a medication which is called an ACE inhibitor, and which improves the heart's performance; I've underlined some of the more interesting ones:

Common side effects of Ramipril Oral:

Joint Pain, Head Pain, Cough

Infrequent side effects of Ramipril Oral:

Abnormally Low Blood Pressure, *Feeling Faint, Dizzy, Rash, Angina, Sensation of Spinning or Whirling, Low Energy, Taste Problems,* Feel Like Throwing Up, *Throwing Up, Diarrhea*

Rare side effects of Ramipril Oral:

Intestinal Angioedema, Head and Neck Angioedema, Allergic Reaction causing Inflammation of Blood Vessels, Blood Pressure Drop Upon Standing, *Vocal Cord Swelling, Pneumonia* with High Amount of Eosinophil White Blood Cells, *Liver Failure, Hepatitis* caused by Drugs, *Yellowing of Skin* or Eyes from Bile Flow Problems, Acute Inflammation of the Pancreas, *Acute Kidney Disease, Blistering Skin* Diseases, Erythema Multiforme, Toxic Epidermal Necrolysis, Stevens-Johnson Syndrome, *Fever,* Abnormal Liver Function Tests, *Giant Hives,* High Amount of Potassium in the Blood, Hemolytic Anemia, *Life Threatening Allergic Reaction,* Acquired Decrease of All Cells in the Blood, *Anemia,* Decreased Blood Platelets, Deficiency of Granulocytes a Type of White Blood Cell, Decreased Neutrophils a Type of White Blood Cell, Disease of the Nerves, *Problems with Eyesight,* Acute *Infection of the Nose, Throat or Sinus, Dry Mouth, Indigestion,* Incomplete or *Infrequent Bowel Movements, Inability to have an Erection,* Sun-*Sensitive Skin, Seizures,* Chronic *Trouble Sleeping, Flu-Like Symptoms, Loss of Appetite, Trouble Breathing, Difficulty Swallowing, Stomach Cramps, Anxious*

Hmm—pain, dizziness, diarrhea, yellow skin, blisters, bad eyesight, no erection, stomach cramps, giant hives! Is it any wonder that the final item is "anxious"?

And these are only a few of the possible side effects from this one medication. Let me mention a couple of the more interesting potential side effects of my other medications: sexual problems, hallucinations, gangrene, confusion, nightmares, hair loss, weight gain, gas, numbness and tingling, burning stomach, cataracts, paralysis of the eye muscles, depression, enlarged breasts, itching, loss of memory, blurred vision, nervous, severe headache, loss of appetite, altered interest in having sexual intercourse.

These are not the types of side effects I thought I was risking when the doctor prescribed the medications. I assumed that the side effects were things like occasional dizziness, occasional nausea, a runny nose—now you're telling me I could get gangrene? With enlarged breasts? And giant hives? Well, with the paralyzed eyes I won't even be able to see any of it!

Let me tell you the reality of side effects, at least for me. I have been taking various heart medications for over 26 years. Not every potential medication you may take, but I have taken ACE inhibitors, Beta blockers, cholesterol lowering drugs, blood thinners, etc.—most of the categories of drugs you are likely to encounter. Have I ever had a *major* side effect? Not really. Have I ever had any side effect? Hard to say.

Why "hard to say"? Because in the last 26 years I have had some dizziness, some muscle pain, occasional headache, flulike symptoms, tingling in the extremities, etc. Are these symptoms a result of the medications taken, or merely a result of other factors in my body, or my environment? That is also "hard to say".

I take a pragmatic approach. If, upon beginning a medication (or shortly thereafter), I begin to experience a negative physical change, I pursue the possibility that the change is a side effect of the medication. However, if I experience something that has been described as a side effect of one of the medications, but have been taking the medication successfully for a period of time, my working hypotheses is that the cause is something other than the medication.

Have I ever had a side effect which has caused me to change medications? The answer is yes, and let me tell you about the two occasions, over a 26-year period. When I was first put on a statin, to help lower my cholesterol, I experienced some stomach discomfort, some bloating—the cardiologist asked me to continue for a week and see if the discomfort subsided, which it did not. He then changed me to a different statin, which I have been using successfully ever since (over a decade), and causes none of that discomfort.

I also had the experience of finding bruises on my body, on my arms and legs primarily. I hadn't bumped into things or injured myself in any way that I could recall, but there were bruises. The bruising actually was the side effect of a medication; the dosage was adjusted, and the bruising stopped.

Now let me tell you about the one side effect of all the drugs I take—I AM ALIVE 26 YEARS LATER!!!! That is it, I am alive. Is that worth a little bit of bloating, and a little bit of bruising—you betcha! So when people ask me if there are any side effects from the medications I've been taking for decades, my answer is always the same, "I'M ALIVE!"

What are the medications that you are likely to be taking?

> **Nitroglycerin**. If, like me, you were rushed to the hospital with a myocardial infarction (heart attack), then you are probably already familiar with nitroglycerin. Nitroglycerin dilates the veins and arteries in the body, which lets the blood flow more easily. It dilates *all* the veins and arteries—so the most common side effect is a splitting headache. You may be prescribed nitroglycerin pills, to carry with you, if you experience angina—the idea here being that if you have an attack of angina, you self-administer the nitroglycerin (by placing one under the tongue), in hopes of getting relief.
>
> Generally, nitroglycerin is not prescribed for daily use, but there are occasions where it may be. If that is the case, it is prescribed as a "patch" that you put on your skin. It is absorbed through the skin throughout the day (and I can tell you from personal experience, it will ensure you have a splitting headache round-the-clock). I used nitro patches for about two years, switched cardiologists when I moved, and had the new cardiologist look at me like I was crazy and ask me why I was wearing a nitro patch. My answer, "My doctor prescribed it". I was unceremoniously informed that, "These patches don't do

anything, you don't need it, stop using it". So much for the medical community all agreeing on a treatment protocol, eh?

Statins—statins are really wonder drugs. They lower cholesterol. So does a watching what you eat—but most people simply are not good about watching what they eat. Also, for a patient who remains vigilant about their eating, the statin will lower cholesterol even further. I have been told by cardiologists, anecdotally, that statins have changed the face of cardiac medicine—that 20 years ago the life of a cardiologist was dominated by responding to one heart attack after another. I'm told that now that statins are in general use for everyone considered high risk, the actual incidence of heart attacks is considerably less than what it was 20 years ago, and on average the size of the heart attacks and the extent of damage done is substantially less than it was years ago. You will most likely be prescribed a statin.

Aspirin—is also a wonder drug. And if you were ever curious, it was actually patented by Bayer, around 1900, and even at that time it was lauded as a wonder drug. You will most likely be prescribed aspirin—the only thing to remember here is you want to take the enteric form, which does not dissolve in your stomach but dissolves further down the digestive tract.

ACE inhibitors—you may be prescribed an Ace inhibitor, which also dilates arteries and makes it easier for the heart to pump blood. It does this without splitting your head open like nitroglycerin.

Beta blockers—these block the effects of adrenaline, and keep your heart pumping at a slower rate than it would if it were affected by the normal workings of adrenaline. Much like statins and food, this doesn't mean you should rely solely on the beta blocker; you will have a better result if you can control your excitement, stress and anger.

60

Whatever medications are prescribed, take them regularly, on time. They are designed to provide maximum benefit when there's a steady supply in your body; they will not work well, and may even be dangerous, in irregular dosages.

You need to understand the benefit derived from each of your medications. Will any of them have potential side effects? Yes, of course. Discuss these with your doctor (but know, right up front, your doctor believes that the benefits far outweigh the potential risks, or he would not be prescribing it). Ask the doctor if there's any ongoing testing that is required for the medication.

Develop a way to ensure you are taking your meds consistently, on time. Most of these meds are designed to have an effect on the heart, either through pressure, or heart rate—so it is imperative that the levels be consistent. I speak from experience when I say— if you miss dosages, figuring out what to take, and when, can become a real mess. Worse yet (and I've done this too), taking the wrong med at the right time is scary—or even worse is taking a pill then realizing or thinking that you're not sure exactly what pill you took. This has led me to organizing my meds into weekly pill containers, and sticking to a rigid schedule—and being aware of what I am taking.

Make sure you understand your meds. After all, you are the person most affected by, and most interested in, your meds; if you don't manage your meds, who will?

I need to take my meds.
Consistently—every day, same time.
My life depends on it.

Back to Work

You might assume after six months of rest and relaxation, I would be anxious to get back to work. Nothing could be further from the truth.

I had become spoiled by having so much time off. This hadn't happened . . . well . . . ever before. Even summer vacations, once I reached 8th grade, involved working a job. I knew this wasn't going to happen again; I didn't want it to end.

And I was nervous about going back; I always thought I was indispensable in my little part of the world, but apparently the place continued running in my absence. I did hear from coworkers occasionally during my absence, but they were careful to avoid discussing stressful issues, so I really had no idea what was going on.

Oddly, through my entire absence, I never had a visit from my boss—odd, because the office was only five minutes from my home, I thought we were close, and I thought we were friends. But his behavior reminded me of the way my Dad's fair-weather friends behaved during his illness; these are the times that reveal your true friends.

When I eventually showed up at work everyone went out of their way to treat me nicely. No one wanted to cause me any stress. Of course, everyone knew I'd had a heart attack—and, regardless what the actual factors affecting me, everyone believed stress was the cause.

But the reality is, heart attack or not, I still had to perform the same as before. Yes, I made some adjustments to staff, and hired an excellent second-in-command to assist me. Regardless, the same stresses that existed before my heart attack were still there upon my return. (And regardless of good intentions, people's ability to insulate me from stress lasted for only a short while—after all, they were obligated to do their jobs, and they needed me to do mine.)

At some point I came to the realization that I couldn't really control the situation, or situations—all I could control is myself. Or, another way to say it is—I may not be able to control everything that happens around me, but I can control the way I react.

Naturally, everyone expected me to act the same way as before, but having a completely new perspective, my actions and responses were different. Different than what they were in the past, and different than what my coworkers had come to expect from me.

My perspective on what was actually important was dramatically different than before. Things that were a very big deal before now seemed like molehills—after all, I have looked death in the eye. I understood that mortality is a really big thing, and a glitch at work, though inconvenient, really isn't—not anymore.

Additionally, I told myself I was not going to let the small things needlessly excite me. I'd been told that stress is a killer. And I was not going to allow those things that, prior, made my blood boil, get me needlessly excited. After all, none of them were worth dying over, or even worth getting sick over.

The way I was reacting and the way I was interacting with people may well have made them feel as though I was a "different person".

(Worth repeating)
RELAX.
Most upsetting things are really not
"life and death", and not worth getting stressed.

And the changes they saw in my professional behavior didn't even include the "lifestyle" changes. Things like exercise and what I eat really can't be put aside; they must be dealt with, even at work.

I was not doing things like drinking sugary sodas, eating potato chips, or even going to fast food restaurants for lunch. While everyone else was scarfing down pizza and soda, I was off somewhere in the supermarket, at a salad bar, trying to find something that wouldn't clog my arteries. Or maybe packing my own lunch.

Which eventually had people making comments like "We should all eat like Stu, it would be better for everyone", or, "Let's all go to the salad bar on Friday". The reality is, the number of people that actually followed up and changed their eating habits as a result of my health situation is pretty small; people really don't seem to get it, not until they have a problem of their own. The other interesting thing is, these comments made me feel very distant from my colleagues. While it was really no one's intent, the comments along with the self-imposed regimen made me feel different, isolated.

My new perspective caused other behavioral changes. When folks said things like, "Let's stop for happy hour after work", my first thought was, "What the heck will I be able to eat or drink?" Not that I wanted to be intentionally rude, or antisocial, but some things that worked fine for me before were now nothing more than unwanted temptations.

I also must find time to exercise daily, regardless of my work schedule. This manifests in things like trying to ride my bike to work, or trying to walk places even though other people drive. During my lunch break, I tried to go for walks—again, comments like "We should all..." And yes, it's one more thing that made me feel apart from my colleagues.

My first trip to New Orleans

Coincidentally the week I returned to work was the industry's annual ATM conference, and that year it was going to be in New Orleans. I was asked to attend, but was nervous about traveling. Suppose something went wrong? Were there good doctors in New Orleans? Did I really want to put myself in a position where I might be in a hospital so far from my family? On the other hand, I had never been to New Orleans, it sounded pretty interesting, and I couldn't spend the rest of my life in a cocoon. So off I went.

I had never been to the ATM convention before. This particular convention attracted bankers from all over North America, bankers who were interested in developing their ATM systems. And at that particular time, the late 1980s, the acceptance and deployment of ATMs still presented huge potential. So thousands attended. The convention was similar to many industry conventions—a big exhibit hall in the convention center where vendors showed their wares, concurrent sessions where industry experts shared their knowledge, individual meetings and private parties. The first evening, there was a cocktail reception—for entertainment at the reception the convention brought in The Temptations to sing their hit songs.

It was a chance to meet with colleagues, make new friends, and come away with more industry information. Also, like most conventions, it was a big party. And here I was, at this big party, with all kinds of eating and behavioral restrictions. While most people were still in bed at 7 a.m., recovering from the night before, I was walking the streets of New Orleans—and I don't mean crawling from pub to pub; I was walking briskly up and down the streets, striving for my target heart rate. While most people were downing their chicory coffee and beignets, I was in my room heating up oatmeal. While most people were just getting warmed up at 10 p.m., and heading out to private parties, I was heading to bed.

I know I was doing the right things, the necessary things, but once again I was feeling very apart from my colleagues. The most disturbing memory of the trip was when one of the other vice presidents invited all eight of our group to "Brennan's for breakfast"; she said it was a New Orleans tradition, and something we absolutely must do. I didn't give it a second thought, knowing that any place that had breakfast food would have something suitable for me—oatmeal, cornflakes, whole-wheat toast, etc.

So we went to Brennan's the final morning of the trip, and were seated at a large round table replete with white linen, beautiful silverware, set amid the beautiful decor. Waiters and busboys in starched white linen jackets and black ties. Very elegant!

When they gave me the menu, I knew I was in trouble. Every page was filled with the richest, creamiest concoctions you could imagine. AND, there was nothing that looked like any breakfast food I had ever eaten! This was a breakfast menu that lacked any traditional eggs, cereal, oatmeal, toast, pancakes . . . .

The menu looked like:

OYSTERS BENEDICT
Fresh Gulf oysters fried to perfection and served on Canadian bacon with Hollandaise sauce.

SHRIMP SARDOU
Deliciously spicy fried shrimp atop sliced artichoke bottoms nestled in a bed of creamed spinach and covered with Hollandaise sauce.

EGGS PORTUGUESE
Flaky pastry shells filled with freshly chopped tomatoes sautéed in butter with parsley and shallots. Topped with poached eggs and covered with Hollandaise sauce.

EGGS NOUVELLE ORLÉANS
Poached eggs served on a bed of lump crabmeat topped with a brandy-cream sauce.

Delicious, eh? Who eats oysters and shrimp and crabmeat for breakfast? Creamed spinach, yum! And let's not forget the Hollandaise, butter and cream. And let's fry it, and throw in some bacon! So, after determining that there was absolutely nothing on the menu that I could eat, I asked the waiter what they had that was consistent with what I could eat.

Now, keep in mind this was 1987, and neither restaurants nor supermarkets catered to the culinary needs of people with health issues in those days. Today, of course, they would whip up some egg whites and come up with a veggie omelet . . . but not 26 years ago!

The only thing they could find in their kitchen, that I was willing to eat, was a rice cake. That's it, a rice cake. So while my colleagues luxuriated in an extravagant breakfast, I got a cup of decaf coffee, and a rice cake with grape jelly.

To this day, it disturbs me. I don't think it was because I couldn't eat the great breakfast, it was more about not being able to do something that the rest of the group could. Over time, I have not only accepted the fact that I can't do some of the things that other people can, I have actually embraced the reality that some of the things I am doing are more healthy, more sensible, and more appropriate than what other people are doing. But at that time, it just made me feel different, alone, like an outsider.

Am I Still The Same Person?

I felt as though I was different from everyone else, partially because I was now unable to participate in certain activities, and partially because I was thinking differently.

Everything that was required of me personally and professionally before the heart attack was still required. But suddenly I had the added burden of managing my nutrition and dedicating adequate time to exercise. I had to prioritize; there are only so many hours in a day, and they must be dedicated to what is most important. Even though I didn't like it, eating properly and exercise were at the top of the list—I knew that otherwise my health would suffer and the rest wouldn't matter.

My daily activities changed. Though exercise took only about an hour, when you consider how much "free time" there is in each day, an hour is a lot. There was also time devoted to food; not just eating, but shopping or preparing. When the use of both fast food and prepared food is eliminated, the amount of time involved in preparing meals increases.

So some of my other activities would need to be de-prioritized. This isn't something I did consciously, and it really wasn't until about five or six years later that I realized exactly what I de-prioritized. I didn't notice all along, but years later I started to think about two specific activities, chess and reading.

From the time I was about 10 years old I had a fascination with chess. I was never really that strong a tournament player, but I was very interested, participated in my local chess club, achieved tournament director status with the United States Chess Federation, and attended weekly meetings of our club. About six years later I realized I had never played another game of chess after my heart attack; never even thought about it.

Prior to the heart attack I was a voracious reader. As extreme as it may sound, one year I spent my entire vacation reading "The

Hobbit", followed by "The Lord of the Rings" trilogy; except for meals and sleep, I never got off the sofa that entire vacation. J.R.R. Tolkien took me on a 2,000-page journey into Middle-earth, and I loved it! Odd as it may sound, about five years after the heart attack I realized I had not read a book—not any book.

I realized it was the time that I had been devoting to chess and reading that I was now devoting to new priorities. I didn't have a desire to get back to chess, but I was concerned at my lack of reading. So I found an interesting, easy book, "The Ragman's Son", the autobiography of Kirk Douglas, the son of dirt poor Jewish immigrants who became a major Hollywood star. While I have never returned to the intensity of my pre-heart attack reading, I do read again.

I think that, subconsciously, I gave up these activities as a result of their passive nature. I came away from the heart attack with an attitude that every day must be lived to the fullest; and to me that means in an active way. Both reading and chess, though they stimulate the mind and sharpen mental acuity, are solitary passive activities—I believe that, subconsciously, I decided this is not the way I wanted to spend the rest of my precious life.

But the change went much deeper than just a couple activities. My approach to time management, and to life itself, to what was important and what was not, had been completely altered.

There hasn't been a single day since the heart attack that I have not thought about the momentary nature of life, the reality that I may not be here long, that it may end at any time, suddenly. Though I may be the same person, with the same personality, I knew that I had to maintain a discipline that had not been part of my prior life. I also knew that I had to focus on only those things that I consider important, to ignore other distractions, and to get things done . . . now.

I really was a changed person. Some people liked the change; others did not. Like it or not, I am different than I was . . . and there's no going back.

Cardiac Cripple?

For a long time after my release from the hospital the slightest twinge was a serious concern to me.

About two weeks prior to the heart attack, I was working on my motorcycle in the garage. I bent over to lift something, something heavy. As I lifted it I got an intense pain in my chest; I mean intense, scary intense. The kind of pain that had me think "OMG, my heart!"

I'm not the kind of person who goes running to the doctor every time I get a sniffle or a muscle spasm. In this case the intensity was something I had never felt before, and it scared me; I placed a call to my family doctor, who had known me for years. When I told him of the pain he said something like, "Stu, don't worry about it. You're just not a candidate for a heart attack. Whatever you lifted was too heavy". Two weeks later I had a heart attack.

In my mind, I related the two events—the pain in the chest, the subsequent heart attack. So post-heart attack any little pain in or near my chest concerned me. If I had a pain, off I went to the doctor—the same doctor, I might mention. I don't know how often I did this, but he always examined me, told me that recovery might be a slow process, small pains were natural, and told me not to worry.

One day, though, he looked me in the eye and said something completely different, "You have a decision to make. Are you going to be a cardiac cripple, or not?" I told him I had never heard that term before. He explained that some people become so consumed with the health of their heart that they interpret every pain, every change, as heart related and potentially life threatening . . . or perhaps as a precursor of some future life-threatening cardiac event. He explained that their obsessive worry effectively turns them into cripples.

70

He went on, "You know, we all have bad days. Even cardiac patients. Sometimes it's just a bad day, not a decline in your health." He was basically telling me to "suck it up", and stop worrying about every little pain. In hindsight, it was good advice . . . great advice. I have known people who, once they started experiencing cardiac problems, made a very big deal out of every little pain. I have seen people with symptoms no worse than my own decide that they should be symptom free—which leads to repeat visits to the cardiologist, repeat tests, multiple stents, and even open-heart surgery.

My grandfather, who was both a doctor and a man with great common sense, also told me something I have never forgotten. At the time I was 24 and he was 72. I had hurt my back, had multiple surgeries to remove herniated discs, and was continuing to experience back problems. Which led to repeat doctor visits, additional diagnostic tests, new medications. And could have, I'm sure, led to more surgeries.

He said "Ya know, I hurt my back when I was your age. It still hurts. Stu, once you have a back problem you're going to always have a back problem". Over the years I learned the truth of his wisdom—I haven't known anyone who's ever had a back problem who hasn't had recurrences. But I've noticed the people with the most serious problems are those who don't recognize the chronic nature of the condition, or their continued vulnerability, and don't care for it or take preventative measures. It seems to me that having a cardiac condition is the same; you must be realistic about having it forever, and vigilant in caring for it.

Scaling the Grand Canyon

A few years after the heart attack, I was feeling some discomfort. Not serious, but real. I was breaking into sweats every time I exercised; but much earlier and easier than normal. And I had this strange uncomfortable feeling that radiated up into my throat. Only when exercising. A common symptom of blockage in an artery is pain when exercising, in the chest or back, or radiating into the arms or throat . . . which subsides when the heartbeat returns to normal. Which mine did. It wasn't horrible, but it was there.

Two possibilities . . . go to the doctor, or wait and see. Normally, I would have gone to the doctor, but my future wife, Rashmika, and I were planning a motorcycle trip in a few days and I knew the doctor would have me in the hospital for an angiogram if he heard these symptoms. I figured the symptoms weren't that bad, only occurred when exercising, so I would go on the trip . . . and take it easy . . . and call the doctor upon my return.

Off we went, to the Grand Canyon . . . of Pennsylvania. About a 5 hour ride, through the Delaware River Water Gap and across the beautiful Endless Mountains of northern Pennsylvania. We left in the morning, but meandered, stopping along the way for lunch, for ice cream (I had frozen yogurt), and to check into the hotel.

We arrived at the Grand Canyon at about 4 p.m. on a beautiful summer day. It's actually a gorge, a very large gorge, which stretches over 45 miles and has depths as great as 1,500 feet. It is very different from "the" Grand Canyon; the GC of PA is beautiful, lush and green, and is not nearly the size of "the" Grand Canyon. We were at the northern end of the gorge, looking down into the canyon, and noticed a sign, "Turkey Path", which indicated a trail leading to the floor of the canyon.

The sign also said "WARNING! As sections of this trail are narrow, steep and hazardous, proper footgear should be worn". We started down, wearing our motorcycle boots of course. It was a gentle decline, a "switchback" trail which descended up and back across the face of the mountain into the gorge. After walking for a long time we encountered folks coming up, and I inquired whether we were near the bottom—they laughed. A little further on we ran into the sign, which read "You are now halfway. Think about how far you have come before proceeding." Big deal, on we went.

Eventually, after descending over a mile of switchbacks, we reached the canyon floor, and that is what was there . . . the floor. Dirt, trees, leaves. I looked up, and could no longer see the sun overhead. "Hmm," I thought, "must be starting to set." Not a very attractive proposition, being at the bottom of this canyon after sundown. Did I mention there were no lights on the trail? No park rangers? No flashlight? No cellphone (early 90s)? We needed to get out of there, and we needed to do it before the sun set, or we would probably be stuck there until morning. I envisioned us huddled together, shivering.

We started up the trail immediately. The first five minutes was fine, then I realized that the gentle switchback trail wasn't really so gentle . . . going up. Matter of fact, it was already starting to feel steep. Now since then, I've done the math, and that switchback trail climbs at a 15 percent grade; next time you encounter a serious hill in your vehicle, the kind of hill that has warning signs indicating the grade for trucks, check it out. I think you'll find a 15 percent grade is serious.

As we're climbing I'm thinking about pacing myself, and keeping proper posture. But my breathing is becoming labored, and I'm starting to sweat. Rashmika, who is always cold, is behind me and is starting to complain that her leather jacket, which she is now carrying, is too heavy (yes, even though it's summer, and more than 70 degrees, she is wearing a heavyweight motorcycle leather jacket). So I grab her jacket, and throw it over my shoulder.

Driven by fear of being stuck after dark, we climbed that trail vigorously. Sweating, breathing hard, legs aching. A 15 percent grade that goes on for a mile is serious; much much more serious than anything I did in my daily life, and much more serious than anything ever thrown at me in a stress test. I was probably well beyond my target heart rate, and for a long time. We collapsed when we got to the top.

Before leaving for the trip, I had never mentioned to Rashmika the discomfort I was feeling. (Matter of fact, she never knew of it until she read this book.) But lying on the ground after that climb, I realized I was feeling none of the symptoms which concerned me. Felt fine the next morning and thereafter. The Grand Canyon challenged me with a much greater stress test that the doctor would have; my fears were quelled. Whatever the symptoms I felt, I knew they weren't coming from my heart.

I'm not saying to ignore obvious symptoms and jeopardize your health; what I am saying is every little pain is not related to your heart. You can't make your heart disease disappear, but you can decide whether you'll spend the rest of your life as a cardiac cripple.

**A heart condition is not going to stop me
from living my life; there is a way.**

Coping with Limitations

What can I do, and what can't I do? How hard can I push myself? How much is too much? What will happen if I push too hard?

The real problem here is finding the limit, and pushing right up to it, but not beyond. On one side, there is the fear that pushing too hard will result in a short-term problem (angina, pain), or a long-term problem (heart attack). On the other side is the necessity to exercise the cardiovascular system, as well as your muscles and joints, as failing to do so will result in further degradation of heart function and general health.

In addition to the invasive diagnostic tests, the doctor also had me do a conventional stress test and a nuclear stress test. During the conventional stress test the doctor had me walk on a treadmill, and as the test progressed, the speed and the incline of the treadmill increased and the doctor observed me, asked how I felt, but kept increasing the speed and the incline. And this is how a stress test goes—at a point, you tell the doctor you've had it, you can't do anymore, and that is the end of the test.

There can be many results—you can have a problem during the stress test, feel pain or discomfort, which would cause the doctor to stop the test at that point. But if everything goes well, and it usually does, you merely walk or jog until you can't anymore, and the test ends.

After the test, the doctor pulled out a chart and told me how many "METs[3]" of exercise I had performed. And the number of METs you can do is a guideline for your daily activities. The chart shows various activities, and whether your heart is strong enough to perform them—things like walking at a slow pace, climbing

---

[3] METs (Metabolic Equivalents) are used for expressing the energy cost of a physical activity as a multiple of the resting metabolic rate. METs are the calculated to determine how much exercise is tolerated during a stress test.

stairs, walking at a faster pace, jogging, walking a golf course, carrying golf clubs, riding a bicycle, etc. It also shows more strenuous activities like running, cross-country skiing, etc.

I didn't appreciate how lucky I was, at the time, when the doctor told me I had performed eight METs. This meant I was able to do everything up to and including rowing, canoeing, kayaking vigorously, dancing vigorously, certain exercise equipment, jogging, downhill skiing, cross-country skiing, carrying heavy objects (100 pounds), and almost every occupation you could think of.

It meant that I didn't have to give up anything physical that I was already doing—hey, my idea of a good time was riding my motorcycle, reading science fiction, watching TV or spending time around the house. I wasn't really looking to be able to climb the Matterhorn, compete in the Ironman or bench press my body weight. So, luckily, from a practical perspective, I really had no physical limitations on exercise, but there were other limitations.

Things like—don't be out in the cold too long, it will affect your heart. Definitely definitely do not be out in the heat too long, it will affect your heart. Do not "overdo" it—whatever it is (shoveling a little snow for five minutes is not a problem, but starting to shovel, and feeling good, and pressing on for 45 minutes could be a serious problem). And, of course, there were guidelines for healthy eating.

Riding to THE Grand Canyon

Let me tell you about one of the "activities" that really challenged some of my limitations. In the mid-90s, Rashmika and I decided to go on a cross-country motorcycle trip with our friends, Tom and Lucille. The general plan was to head west. We would spend the first night in Pittsburgh, visiting our son, then continue toward the southwest, eventually reaching the Grand Canyon. We would then take a different route back across the United States. In August.

One of the initial things I did was visit my cardiologist. She was an extremely sharp, talented, caring doctor, and I valued her opinion. I told her the plan, and asked her advice—her reply,

"Don't go". When I pushed harder for suggestions, she kept giving me the same answer, "Don't go". She stopped short of saying, "You'll die" (but I could tell that's what she was thinking). I was not deterred.

Doctors are very cautious, and they don't always understand your priorities.

Next stop, general practitioner Dr. David George, a doctor with an old-fashioned approach to medicine. He was very pragmatic, and was just as willing to use tried-and-true home remedies as he was to prescribe modern medications. His response was very different. He advised me to make sure I stayed fully hydrated throughout the trip, and do my best to avoid excessive heat — actually, he suggested riding in the early morning and at night. This made me feel better; at least he wasn't reacting as though it was going to be a one-way trip.

When I got home, I went to work on solving the hydration problem. I mounted bicycle water bottle cages on top of the saddlebags of my Harley-Davidson, so that while riding I could easily grab a water bottle. Hey, if it worked for Greg LeMond on his 2,000-mile Tour de France win, it should work for me. I just had to remember to do it.

The first night of the trip we arrived in Pittsburgh as planned; when I watched the weather report I saw the temperature in Arizona, near the Grand Canyon, was 112 degrees. So we modified our route a bit, and headed due west to New Philadelphia, Ohio, where we visited Warther's cutlery and museum, where they still today make some of the finest cutlery in the world, using the same methods and materials they did 100 years ago.

The next day we wound up at Conner's Prairie, sort of a Midwestern farm town version of Williamsburg, Virginia; the town was of course not air conditioned, and was sweltering. By the third night we were in Peoria, Illinois; the temperature reported at the Grand Canyon had risen to 117 degrees.

So we continued west, but moved slightly north. By the next afternoon we were in Ames, Iowa; believe it or not, by 1 p.m. it was 105 degrees in Ames. We headed for a local mall, where we sat in the air-conditioning and took in a movie.

Though we kept checking the weather reports every night, we never saw the temperature drop in Arizona, so we continued west and slightly north, eventually arriving in Sturgis, South Dakota. Sturgis is the home of the largest motorcycle rally in the world, but we were actually a week early (not a surprise, as we never really intended to be there at all). We had a great time in Sturgis, hanging out with all the vendors as they pulled in to set up. We also got to see the amazing sights of the Dakotas and Wyoming—Devils Tower, the Black Hills, the Crazy Horse Memorial, Mount Rushmore, the Badlands. At one point, we shared a small, narrow road with a buffalo that dwarfed us, towering over Rashmika, me, and our Harley.

And let me mention, the trip did not prevent doing the other things necessary for my health. I was able to still eat carefully everywhere we went. I exercised every day—I was up every morning early, and took my daily walk before breakfast. Actually, Lucy was recovering from a health issue, and also wanted to exercise to get back in shape. So many mornings I had company on my walk, and it was a great way to start the day.

Still trying to stay out of the heat, we decided to make our return trip in the north, so we crossed the most northern states and eventually got to the other side of the Great Lakes, entering Canada at Sault Ste. Marie. We rode east across Canada, took a ferry boat across Lake Huron, rode through Toronto, and eventually came back into the United States at Niagara Falls. Even though we never made it to the Grand Canyon (the one in the southwest), this was one of the most memorable trips ever. Four thousand miles outdoors filled with buffalo, prairie dogs, mountain sculpture, motorcycles, and the beauty and majesty of America.

It's not about the Destination, it's about the Journey.

Had I followed the advice of the cardiologist, a woman who I truly trusted, it would never have happened. Am I suggesting that you not follow the advice of your doctor—no! What I am suggesting is this—know your doctor, and know yourself. I have not known many cardiologists, but the ones I have all have something in common—they err on the side of caution. I suppose this is because the decisions they make can be life or death, and neither they, nor any reasonable person, is going to advise another person to take risks which could be deadly.

Somewhere between the cardiologists' cautious point of view of what is acceptable, and living a totally unrestrained uninhibited life, most likely lies the reality of what you can do. Had Rashmika and I completely ignored pragmatist Dr. George's advice, and followed our original plan to ride to the Grand Canyon, where the daily highs were exceeding 110 degrees, it may have indeed been a one-way trip for me. But taking some reasonable steps to ensure I didn't exceed limitations allowed me to have one of the great adventures of my life.

The limitations of heart disease could have sentenced me to a life of indoor living, modest amounts of activity, and being forced to live vicariously through TV, books, and the experiences of others. In fact, being realistic and appropriately cautious has allowed me to live a full and interesting life.

part three
a new life

Major Changes

Though the changes I needed to make for food, exercise and stress were dramatic, there were actually much more significant changes that resulted from the realization of my mortality.

When you have a life threatening event, be it a heart attack, car accident, whatever, the implications of that event are initially in the forefront of your mind, but slowly fade. Which is why so many people react to events like heart attack by walking the straight and narrow—watching what they eat, exercising regularly—but eventually, as the fear fades, start to backslide. A little less exercise, a little more dessert. Until eventually, they are right back where they began.

Not so in my case—from the night Dr. Levin told me, "We will see", I have never forgotten death could come any time, and in my case, could come unexpectedly and without warning. So the notion that I had plenty of time to do the things I wanted, or to accomplish the things that I thought were important, dissolved in the year following the heart attack. From that time forward I have been driven to get things done, because I fear that if I don't do them now. . . .

There were three aspects of my life that bore no resemblance to what I once imagined would be the perfect life for me:

Marriage
Career
Where I lived

Actually, the major components of my life. Combined, it was a problem, a huge problem. At 37, was I ready to throw in the towel, and continue to drift down the river of life? Or was I going to jump off the boat, swim through alligators and sharks to the distant shore, and set off in another direction?

We've all seen these lists of "life events" that cause stress— death of a parent, loss of your job, etc. And certain things rank very high on that list. Things like . . . divorce. Moving. New job. The very things I needed—but not just one of them, all three. Regardless that I had a major heart attack, and was supposed to avoid stress, these changes needed to be made. If I died suddenly I would have died regretting that I never tried to live the life I wanted, that I had allowed others to set my direction, that I had just drifted through life taking the easy way out.

So, knowing that the stress involved in major change was a serious risk that had to be controlled, I set out to change to course of the rest of my life.

Marriage / Divorce

When I was young I read books about exotic places, brave men and women, great deeds. I always wanted to be in those places, doing those deeds—but instead I was in my little town, with my nose in a book. I wasn't very good athletically, didn't have the kind of good looks that girls liked, and to top it all off I was painfully shy. I was a loner, never quite fitting in.

When I was 16, I met a beautiful girl; I never knew why, but she really liked me. And I liked her. She had a nice personality, and a great sense of humor. And did I mention she was beautiful? Through the lens of hindsight I can now tell you we had nothing in common—hobbies, interests, friends—nothing. But at the time it didn't seem to matter; when you're young and in love those things are not obvious, or relevant.

When I was 17, in the mid-60s, I discovered drugs. Marijuana use was rampant through kids my age. I tried it; it seemed to relax me. I became part of a clique; we were all bonded through the secrecy that comes with illegal drug use.

Then I discovered "speed". This was like a magical elixir to someone who suffered painful shyness; on speed I had no inhibitions about interacting with others. I instantly became an extrovert, and I loved it. Of course, I felt I could control the usage. Eventually though, I was constantly high—either on speed to get through the days, or grass to get settled back down.

A few years later we decided to get an apartment, and move in together. This wasn't the most acceptable thing to do in the '60s, at least not for two kids from "nice families". Our parents immediately went to work convincing us to get married, rather than embarrass the families by "shacking up" (their words). So at 21, this motorcycle-riding, long-haired druggie married his 19-year-old beautiful girlfriend with the nice personality and great sense of humor. Trouble was, we still had nothing in common, except we liked each other.

Within a couple years of marrying, I gave up drugs. Entirely, and for life. Cut all ties to anything to do with the drug culture. People who had been my good friends for several years never saw me again (not to this day). I was never again seen in places I had frequented. Stopped, cold turkey, and never looked back.

As we moved into our mid-20s, we had a baby. A couple years later, we bought a house. Then a second baby. Two children, a mortgage, two cars, PTA meetings, T-ball practice. Living the lives of average middle-class Americans.

But something that never changed was . . . we really had nothing in common, except the life that we had built together. My interests were motorcycles, chess and science fiction; her interests were beauty culture and, well, I don't even know. But I do know that the things I had passion for held no appeal for her. And she really didn't like my motorcycle friends.

The reason I was with friends, not my wife, on that fateful Sunday was that as much as a big biker rally, with Harleys, music, drag races and a swap meet attracted me, it repulsed her. She was relieved that I would go alone, and leave her out of it; I was not. And I was not willing to face the rest of my life with a companion who had no interest in the things that I loved.

When you have a wife and two children, it's not easy to make a change without hurting the ones you love. And it wasn't easy. But my love and my wife's love for the children prevented us from going down a path of hate and destruction. We separated about three years after the heart attack and eventually divorced. Since then we have celebrated at the marriages of our children, have had

Thanksgiving dinner together, and we grandparent together. My ex-wife and I live far apart and see each other rarely; but we remain friends, love each other in a way only we understand, and look forward to those times when we see each other.

Career

Once I put drugs behind me, I needed a job. A real job—steady, respectable, upwardly mobile. Lucky for me, my family knew the people who ran a bank, and arranged an interview. I suddenly had a job in the "coin room" at Guarantee Bank in Atlantic City. Locked up in a little room with bags of coins, counting machines and two other employees.

Before long I got my big break. The morning after the company Christmas party, the assistant branch manager came to work hung over, so hung over he fell asleep in the break room. The branch manager was desperate for someone to man the new accounts desk in the bank lobby and open accounts for new customers. He stuck his head in the coin room, and there was only one person appropriately dressed (jacket and tie); I got my chance!

Apparently I did pretty well, because within a few months I was approached by the Bank's internal auditor who asked if I would like to join the audit staff. A golden opportunity for me to learn banking from Mr. Welch, a retired lawyer and FBI agent, and his brilliant assistant, Bob Tranter. Bob was just a few years older than me, but he had an unbelievable depth of knowledge; the likes of which I never again encountered in my 24 years of banking.

I became a valued member of the audit staff, where I stayed and learned the nuts and bolts of banking for eight years. Then I managed bank security, armored cars, and fraud prevention for a few years. Then on to Bank Operations for a few years. Then Support Services, where I managed the bank's real estate, communications, money rooms and armored cars.

And somewhere in the middle of all that, I took responsibility for ATMs. I was the auditor who wrote all the procedures when we installed our first ATM in 1976. I was the leader of the team that went out on nights and weekends to keep the ATMs running.

I was the manager who bought the armored trucks so we could install ATMs in casinos and colleges. I was the banker who went to Donald Trump's office to discuss putting ATMs in his casinos.

By the time of the heart attack, I was a vice president, managing the ATM business of statewide bank, a job I could do with my eyes closed. Yes, there were challenges, but they were more along the lines of the latest senior management "fire drill" than anything else. But I knew if I could gain access to the Board of Directors in New York City, I could make a real impact on the way the business was being run, on our customers, and on our bottom line.

Four years after the heart attack I drove into my newly assigned space, walked to the edge of the parking deck and, overlooking the Statue of Liberty, gazed straight across the river at the Twin Towers of the World Trade Center. I regretted that my Dad hadn't lived to know that I made it, that I was here, an integral part of the management team of a colossal global bank, at the center, the pinnacle, of the world of banking and finance.

Where I Lived

As a young child, I lived in a suburb of Philadelphia, but when I was nine years old we moved to the Atlantic City, New Jersey area, where my mother's family lived.

Atlantic City was a resort town built in the mid-1800s. The railroads saw an opportunity to create a seaside health resort, and ran a line from Philadelphia right to the Atlantic Ocean. They also built an immense facility, the United States Hotel, which was the largest hotel in the nation, and dropped passengers off at the front door of the hotel. By the mid-1870s the demand was so great that it took two railroads to serve the resort.

The boom continued into the early 20th century; sprawling palatial hotels were built along the Boardwalk, facing the sea. Atlantic City was the home of the Miss America Pageant and salt water taffy. The Steel Pier stretched a quarter mile into the sea, culminating in an open arena where daredevils walked a tightrope, dove hundreds of feet into the sea, and the famous Diving Horse took its daily plunge. And there was, of course, the world famous

Boardwalk, the place to be seen dressed in all your finery. A fabulous seaside resort.

But progress wasn't kind. Returning veterans from World War II had new opportunities, the opportunity to own their own home, and the opportunity to own an automobile. Widespread car ownership in the mid-20th century changed the way people vacationed, no longer limiting them to destinations on the railroads. Motels (motor hotels) sprang up around the nation, and those Philadelphians that prior flocked to "the shore", now found themselves in the Pocono Mountains, the Catskills, and Miami Beach for vacation.

By the time I reached Atlantic City in the late 1950s, those huge hotels, the palaces by the sea, were still open, but were no longer overflowing with the wealthy, the chic. The boardwalk was busy, but the fine shops and auction houses of the past had been replaced with souvenir stores and cut-rate merchants. The amusement piers which stretched into the sea were still open, but the paint was peeling and the rides went half empty. The Boardwalk Empire had fallen. And it only got worse.

One by one, the beautiful hotels closed, bankrupt or foreclosed. The amusement piers closed. The Boardwalk never closed, but the merchants became more and more honky-tonk. Unemployment soared; the percentage of residents collecting unemployment insurance became the highest in the state. And there was no relief for decades.

Growing up in this bankrupt resort area was uninspiring; it was bereft of anything you would call art or culture. There was no theater—not even community theater. There was no symphony or opera. There were, and are, no museums, art or otherwise. There were no professional or semipro sports teams. The fabulous Convention Hall, the largest in the world, was used for the annual Miss America Pageant and some occasional professional wrestling matches; it sat idle most of the year.

One of the things the area did have, and please don't laugh, was cable TV—long before most of the nation. Atlantic City was too far from New York to receive over-the-air TV signal, and just far enough away from Philadelphia to make TV reception "iffy". By the time I arrived in the late 50s there was already cable TV, and we received more channels than even the large cities, because channels from both New York and Philadelphia were piped in.

But how satisfying is life in a place where the most interesting thing you can find is TV? Sure, I played chess on Thursday nights. I read novels. But go to a show? The symphony? Never. Four years after the heart attack I was living 40 minutes from New York, going for walks in Washington Square Park, going to Lincoln Center for the symphony, going to Madison Square Garden for the Westminster Kennel Club Show, going to the Met, to MOMA. The world opened up not just for me, but for those around me.

Do the things that make your life complete.
Do them now.

I didn't know how long I was going to live. I knew I couldn't afford to wait to make fundamental changes. While I had always wanted a change, I never before felt the urgency. I always assumed I'd live to be old, like my grandparents. I always assumed there'd be plenty of time to find whatever I was looking for in life. Suddenly I knew there were no guarantees.

My realization of mortality made me more prepared to change my life than to continue to drift along, taking the easy route. I was driven to make the changes, even understanding the real, significant hurdles that would have to be met. Four years after the heart attack I was living a completely different life, but was maintaining the most important link to my former life, a relationship with my teenage children.

What it really all came down to was, "life is short". Life is too short to delay. We have all heard from older people that life goes by "in the blink of an eye"; of course, that's from older people, and we're always thinking that we are also going to become older people. That doesn't take into account heart attacks, auto accidents, or something else that could cut our life short. The attitude I developed was, I simply could not afford to wait to live my life—if I did, it might never happen.

Finding Good Doctors

I cannot stress enough how important it is to have good doctors. To me, a good doctor is one with excellent medical knowledge and skill, a caring attitude, and (equally important) the ability to work with me.

Dealing with a heart condition requires two doctors, both essential. A GP (general practitioner, or primary care physician), and a cardiologist.

The general practitioner needs to have a comprehensive, almost encyclopedic, knowledge of medicine; because the GP doesn't specialize, he needs a full understanding of all anatomical function and medical conditions so he can properly diagnose any issue, and either provide the care, or get you to specialized care.

The GP also needs to have a good working knowledge of the patient, of those other factors that affect health. So either the GP needs to know you pretty well, or you need to keep the GP informed of relevant factors.

Ideally, the GP is someone who has extensive experience, and still keeps up on the latest medical developments. So, no newbies or has-beens—and please don't misinterpret. I am not suggesting you avoid young or old doctors; there are some young doctors whose training has given them extensive experience, and many older doctors who have retained their passion for knowing the latest developments, techniques and treatments.

The cardiologist will look after the health of your heart. Don't decide you don't need a cardiologist for ongoing care, that your GP can cover it. Your heart, the organ that powers your body, has been compromised, and you need the finest possible care; you need a specialist. This needs to be a doctor who lives and breathes cardiac medicine. Who has a passion for it and its patients. Who is extensively experienced and passionately pursues new knowledge (same as the GP).

The first question on how to find "good doctors" is to ask yourself where you got your current doctors. Most likely your GP is someone who you personally selected, and who was already taking care of your health. If you have developed a heart condition your cardiologist may not be someone who you personally selected—perhaps like me you were rushed to the hospital, saved by a great doctor, and this doctor became your cardiologist. Or perhaps you were experiencing symptoms, and your GP referred you to a cardiologist. So how do you know if these people are really any good?

There is no objective published system of grading for doctors; much like politicians, you are forced to figure it out on your own. Wouldn't it be wonderful if we could review statistics for each doctor? I would love to know about patient turnover, average time per appointment, mortality rate, etc. Unfortunately, it is not tracked or available. The only thing remotely close is the various ratings on the internet, which are allegedly patient feedback; I have found many of these internet ratings (for doctors, restaurants, hotels, etc.) to be extremely inaccurate and misleading, for reasons that could take an entire chapter to explain.

Start with referrals and interviews. Ask friends, neighbors, and other doctors. You are looking for doctors in your own area, and certainly other people you know use doctors, so ask your friends and neighbors. You are currently seeing some doctors; call them, ask them who they recommend, and why (I am most impressed when a doctor recommends someone they use themselves, or send their family to.)

Every time I have moved forward on a referral to a doctor (and I don't mean in an emergency situation) I have made an appointment for the purpose of meeting the doctor. I haven't said, "I want to interview the doctor"; I have said, "I am a new patient and would like to come in and meet the doctor". I have given the office my medical history, and spent the appointment talking to the doctor about the state of my health, and listening to the doctor's responses. It has given us a chance to get started on the right foot—not to say it won't be OK otherwise, but if on your first visit you have laryngitis, or diverticulitis, you may not be in a position or a state of mind to meet and bond with the doctor. Go in first, and talk—most doctors will benefit from that first appointment as much as you will.

Remember what Lincoln said: "You can fool some of the people all of the time, all of the people some of the time, but you cannot fool all of the people all of the time." Point being, if you ask people, and check it out yourself, you will get to the bottom of it.

Then there's the other piece, my need for a doctor who can work with me, who I'm comfortable with, who I'm confident in. We all have different needs when we interact with doctors—some of us need a doctor who will give us detailed medical explanations, some of us need a doctor who will tell us how we will be treated, and some of us need a doctor who exudes confidence and provides no explanations.

First decide what it is you want. The best way to do this is to think about whatever doctor you're currently comfortable with, and what the traits are of that doctor. If you like the detailed explanation he/she gives you, if you like the time he/she spends, if you like the no-nonsense attitude . . . note these things. These are the things you want in a doctor.

I have been very fortunate with doctors over the last several decades. If I consider my heart attack a starting point, I was already seeing a GP that I was very comfortable with. And, by default, Dr. Jack Levin (the cardiologist who saved my life) became my initial cardiologist—lucky for me, he is an excellent physician and a caring person.

But over the years I moved three times to distant locations that required I find new doctors. Prior to every move I asked my current doctors for recommendations—and every one of them took the time to research potential doctors in the new location and gave me excellent recommendations.

There is only one time in all the years that one of these recommendations didn't work out; I went in, met the doctor, and all seemed OK. But after two visits I felt the doctor really wasn't interested. I moved on to the next recommendation, met that doctor, a knowledgeable, caring GP who has helped me manage my health for over twenty years.

I could tell you some other stories about changing doctors. The oncologist my mother was seeing who seemed devoid of any human feeling (I guess it was just his way). The dentist who could never be less than an hour late for an appointment. The dentist who I made an initial appointment with and had me sit in the waiting room over an hour past the appointed time—I got up and left, never even met her.

Next to your immediate family, your doctor may be the most important person in your life. Not your auto mechanic, your hair stylist, or your bookie—your doctor, the person who will help manage your health. If you don't have an excellent relationship with your doctor, one that you are completely confident and comfortable with, then find a new doctor. Don't accept just any doctor you found on the river of life; find doctors who are as interested in your health as you are, who have a "style" you're comfortable with, who you trust, and who you like.

Find the best doctors you can, but accept that you need to manage your own health, no one else can. Not your doctor, not your therapist, not your spouse. You.

Daily Temptations

I have always been tempted by forbidden fruit. Just tell me I can't do it—"You're too young for that movie." "It's too dangerous." ("If all the other kids jumped off a bridge, would you jump off?") "Nice people don't do that." I can't tell you why, but when I heard things like that, it just increased my desire. I made sure I saw the film, read the book, jumped off the bridge, or did whatever it was that the "not nice" people were doing.

Suddenly I'm told that I should not eat certain foods, should not smoke, should avoid certain activities, and should follow completely different protocols. And, deep down, I know this is all good advice, and in my best interest; but I have a history of pushing back, resisting, any suggestions from anyone that I do anything. It took me a while to accept that I needed to do these things, *for myself*. Regardless, not because, others were suggesting them. But once I accepted, I became committed to doing the best I could (within reason). Trouble is, it's not easy.

I ride a motorcycle. Sometimes I'm out riding, minding my own business, with my mind in that zone where it goes whenever I'm on a motorcycle—a state of Zen, where I am one with the motorcycle (and motorcycling is one of those activities where you'd better be able to achieve a state of Zen, because if your mind is elsewhere, the result can be very ugly). And suddenly my senses are assaulted, my Zen is shattered, my attention is diverted—there's a McDonald's! Somewhere within a quarter-mile! The smell is overwhelming! French fries! Big Mac! Vanilla shake!

It happens nearly every time I ride. I can smell a fast food restaurant anywhere in the vicinity. The urge to pull in, order a Big Mac and fries happens every time I ride through that smell. But years ago I read the nutrition information for a Big Mac; if you have a cholesterol problem, or a problem with atherosclerosis, a Big Mac (or a Whopper, Double Stack, sliders, etc.) is literally the "heartstopper special". These things have enough fat to grease the wheel bearings on your car, enough salt and cholesterol to do unimaginable damage to your body.

Movie theaters. The only place you can see the "Lord of the Rings", "Star Trek", "Star Wars", "Lawrence of Arabia", on a big screen. And they've gotten better over the years—with gigantic IMAX screens, comfortable stadium seating, realistic surround sound. Several times a year I go to a theater to see some specific movie that needs to be seen on the big screen. Do I need to even say it? The smell of popcorn! Now, the popcorn is not the problem—but theaters put so much salt on popcorn that if you have any issue with blood pressure, you might as well just make an appointment with the doctor for 30 minutes after you visit the snack stand.

Restaurants. An obvious problem. But they are not a problem because they don't have healthy foods—over the last 20 years the restaurant industry has realized that there are a good percentage of people who need healthy alternatives. The problem is, the items on the menu sound so delectable. How can you possibly walk into the Carnegie Deli, and not order a hot pastrami, on rye, drenched in Russian dressing? How could you possibly visit Philadelphia and not order a Philly cheese steak with fried onions? Would any visit to Chicago be complete without deep dish pizza? And this is only the beginning—everywhere is famous for something!

In the last 20 years, restaurants have added alternatives. Problem is, they may not sound all that appetizing—the "Doctor's Choice Breakfast", consisting of an egg white omelet with tomatoes and onions, a side of cottage cheese, and some dry toast certainly doesn't sound as good as two eggs over easy, home fries, bacon, and a short stack of pancakes.

I've learned you don't need to be limited to the "healthy alternatives" on the menu. If you see an item on the menu, something like fish in a creamy French sauce, on a bed of some kind of vegetables or greens, with some kind of potatoes, have a conversation with your server. Ask whether they can make the same fish without the cream sauce, using olive oil, and some spices—ask them to make the vegetables without butter. You'll be surprised at not only how accommodating they are, but how much pride some kitchens and chefs take in being able to accommodate you.

And then there are desserts. People always seem amazed that I don't eat desserts. When other people are ordering tiramisu, New York cheesecake, black forest cake, pie and ice cream, I just order either decaf coffee or decaf cappuccino. I take, literally, a "taste" (definition of "a taste"—a little bit on the edge of a fork or spoon) of whatever my wife is having. The taste lets me know what it is, and lets me appreciate the dessert—the difference between taking a taste, and eating a dessert, is the difference between appreciating the dessert and clogging my arteries. It's that simple. I get just as much out of "the taste" as I need.

Do I ever "cheat"? There are a few things I try to remember— one is "all things in moderation". As it relates to things that I really should not do, I have modified that to "all things on rare occasions". And let me tell you what some of them are, at least for me:

A rare juicy steak. I am not a vegetarian, and I am not opposed to eating red meat. But on a regular basis I get my "meat" in the form of fish or fowl, and this includes things like burgers (turkey-burgers—made on our grill). But, occasionally, I like a good rare steak—my definition of "occasionally" is on each of my "decade" birthdays, my 50th, 60th, etc. And on those occasions, I want a great steak—so we go to Peter Luger Steakhouse in Brooklyn, arguably one of the great steak houses in the world. The satisfaction lasts me for the next decade.

A great dessert. Every year, or at least every other year, we try to get to Commander's Palace in New Orleans, perhaps the best restaurant in the United States. And they do a fantastic job, cooking me the best meal you can imagine, and doing it every year without any butter, cream, etc. The meal has been so good at times that I have tasted it, called over the waiter, and actually sent it back to the kitchen as, after tasting, I was convinced it was made with butter (which it was not!). But that is not the point—as I said, I don't eat desserts, but my "occasional" dessert is Bananas Foster, a fabulous flambéed dessert of vanilla ice cream, butter, cinnamon, bananas and rum. I have it once a year (unless we don't get to New Orleans that year, in which case it gets skipped), and that is the only dessert I ever have. No more than one dessert a year.

I'm going to take you back to something I said in an earlier chapter, about my solution for smoking. Where I was really struggling with the idea of never being able to smoke again—but I was able to cope with the idea of just not smoking the "next cigarette". Just like they teach people at AA—it's not about giving up drinking forever; it's about not having the next drink.

Same with all the temptations in my path—I just don't eat the "next" dessert, the "next" steak, the "next" French fries, the "next" cigarette, etc. In some cases, the temptation never goes away—but in many cases (and smoking is a good example) after being away from it for long enough, the temptation passes. I no longer have any desire to smoke a cigarette; the smell, which used to be so compelling, no longer attracts me.

And the same is true of many of the things I have given up. Surprisingly, I have found that some things which had no appeal to me prior, have become substitutes for those things that I have given up. I do not walk around daily feeling like I am being denied things I want—my life, and my senses (taste, smell, touch) are being fully satisfied.

The key is accepting that your body has different requirements than before, and breaking familiar habits. Just know, some things may never go away—the smell of a fast food restaurant when I'm zipping down the road is just as attractive today as it was 20 years ago . . . but I'm not stopping for that next burger, that next order of fries.

I can change, I have willpower.
The changes I need are for me, no one else.

Living with Heart Disease

Living with heart disease means living with a slew of tasks and responsibilities you never thought about before. Though my condition may not be exactly the same as your own, let me tell you about some of them.

Medications

I now take medications as part of my daily routine. Before, the only time I took medications were when I was ill or injured — antibiotics, painkillers, etc., as needed. Now I am on a strict schedule for medications at specific times each day.

I have learned, the hard way, not to inadvertently "skip" a dosage—skipping a dosage always leads to the quandary of whether to take the medication late, or skip until the next dose. Which, of course, leaves me wondering if I take the dose late will that result in too great a concentration in my system when I take the next dosage, or if I skip the dose will I be unprotected and subject to a heart problem. So I don't skip.

Initially, it was quite a challenge. I had meds that I took upon awakening, meds at noon, meds at 3 p.m., and meds at dinner. It seemed to always be a problem, either confusing what meds I was supposed to take, or becoming so busy I simply forgot. I took to wearing a wristwatch with the alarm—that helped some. In the end, I just learned to stick to the schedule (and now, thank goodness, I take all my meds upon awakening—except for the statin, just before bedtime).

Doctor Appointments

"Regular" doctors appointments were not part of my life—I felt fine, so I didn't do things like an annual physical, with the exception of regular dental appointments.

With heart disease, there needs to be periodic check-ups of your heart, so the current condition can be compared to "the baseline" (the condition of your heart when the problem began). My cardiologist recommends two or three appointments a year. He does an EKG, listens to my heart, and asks about any symptoms. Based what he sees and hears, he may recommend additional testing (see below).

My increased awareness and concern also led to regular appointments with my primary care physician. I try to go for an annual checkup, for all those other things that a cardiologist is not looking at. Apparently, the older you get the more of those things there are.

In a perfect world the primary care physician and the cardiologist are both informed and sensitive to the treatment that the other is giving you. If they are not, you need to make that happen.

Ongoing Testing
Blood tests

First, there will surely be ongoing blood tests. Regardless whether you are taking a blood thinner or not, there will be regular tests to determine your level of cholesterol.

Most likely, your doctor will want your cholesterol tested annually. A cholesterol test is called a "fasting lipid profile"; this means, surprise, surprise, you need to be fasting. Different labs and different doctors will give you different parameters for the fast. What has worked best for me is to schedule the blood test for as early as the lab can do (and generally the test facilities schedule appointments as early as 7 a.m.); I then fast from dinner the night before, which is about a 12-hour period.

The desired result from your fasting lipid profile is:

- ♥ Overall cholesterol—as low as possible
- ♥ LDL (low-density lipids, this is the "bad cholesterol")—as low as possible
- ♥ HDL (high-density lipids, the "good" cholesterol)—as high as possible.

Based on your results the doctor may recommend a change in medications or foods to decrease your LDL, and a change in your exercise regimen and/or weight to increase your HDL.

Stress tests

The doctor may recommend a stress test on occasion to observe your heart under exercise, as discussed in the chapter "Coping With Limitations".

It is also possible the doctor may occasionally recommend a "nuclear" stress test. This also requires exercise on a treadmill, but includes the injection of a nuclear isotope into your bloodstream (through an IV line in the back of your hand). Following the exercise component, you are placed in a large camera apparatus, which takes a series of photographs of your heart, and produces high definition images of the nuclear isotopes flowing through the arteries of your heart. This allows the doctor to know if there is any ischemia, meaning inadequate supply of blood, to any part of the heart.

Echocardiogram

Another common procedure is the "echocardiogram". This is an ultrasound of the heart, similar to the ultrasounds done on pregnant women. It is not an invasive test; it is done by a technician passing a probe over the walls of your chest. Sound waves are used to produce an image of the heart. The echocardiogram lets the doctor know your "ejection fraction", (the percentage of blood leaving your heart after each contraction); it is a measure of the efficiency of the pumping action of the heart.

Cardiac Angiogram

This is an invasive procedure which is the definitive test for finding blockages and/or narrowing in the arteries of the heart. As mentioned earlier, this is a procedure done in a Cath Lab (sometimes in the hospital, sometimes in a private facility), by a doctor supported by a team of nurses. This is generally done if you are having symptoms that your cardiologist believes are caused by a narrowing, or blockage, in an artery. Often times, the doctor performing the angiogram, and his team, have set up the OR so that if, in fact, a blockage is revealed they can immediately perform a balloon angioplasty, and perhaps also insert a stent in the blocked artery.

Procedures
Angioplasty

Angioplasty involves temporarily inserting and blowing up a tiny balloon where your artery is clogged to help widen the artery. Angioplasty is often combined with the permanent placement of a small wire mesh tube called a stent to help prop the artery open and decrease the chance of it narrowing again.

In my case, I have had three angioplasties over a 26-year period; in two cases stents were inserted to help keep those arteries open. In all three cases, the angioplasties corrected the symptoms of angina I was experiencing when exercising. As a result, I have never required "bypass" surgery.

Bypass Surgery

Bypass is a procedure used to "bypass" blockages in heart arteries. A bypass is created by taking a piece of vein or artery from elsewhere in the body, and grafting it to the affected coronary artery, jumping over the blockage. It is a form of open heart surgery, and requires the chest be opened, and generally requires the heart be stopped and the patient be placed on a heart and lung machine during the surgery.

While bypass is certainly a major surgery, it generally gives the patient a new lease on life. The procedure generally requires four days' hospitalization, and a period of recuperation and rehabilitation at home.

<u>Limitations and precautions</u>

Though all heart patients will be advised to stop smoking, eat correctly and exercise regularly, there are other limitations that may be unique, based on an individual's medical condition, physical condition, interests and abilities. Let me mention a few that affect most heart patients.

What will I eat?

There are many days that I go places and do things that fill the whole day. Sometimes I know exactly what food I will eat—but other times either I know there are no good food options at my destination, or I don't know. In those cases, I take food with me; the easiest things I have found to take are (1) a sandwich of wheat toast, honey and reduced-fat peanut butter (easy to put in a Ziploc sandwich bag), and (2) bananas.

And, for the record, I do not feel at all self-conscious when I pull out my food; my heart health is way more important.

Water—there are many situations where I bring along bottled water.

I bring food and water when I go to events, no-salt pretzels when I go to movies (to resist the popcorn!), and when I travel. The alternatives for food in airports, train stations and on airplanes are very often limited—I am very content to be munching on my peanut butter sandwich and banana when everyone else is grumbling about how the airlines no longer provide food. At biker events I am the strange guy who is not scarfing down burgers, hotdogs and pork; I feel completely at ease enjoying the festivities with my bottled water and bagged lunch.

Temperature extremes.

This is certainly something I never thought about before; if it was cold, I put on more clothing, if it was hot I took off clothing. While this is still true, temperature extremes can be dangerous to someone with heart disease, so extra care must be taken to ensure that one is not subjected to extreme heat, or extreme cold, for too long a period.

Sounds easy. Except that many of us like outdoor activities, like snow skiing, or relaxing on the beach—both activities which could easily expose you to temperature extremes. In my case—motorcycling. Now, most people think of motorcycling as a warm weather activity, which it is—unless you are a diehard like me, and ride 12 months a year in the Northeast of the United States. Many years, I participate with a group called the Polar Bears—from November until April we meet for lunch each Sunday, riding our motorcycles to the meeting spot, which is usually about two hours from home. There are days in February, when the high temperature doesn't exceed 20 degrees Fahrenheit.

Sounds like one of those activities that I would have to give up, right? Being out in temperatures below 20 degrees, for at least four hours, and moving on a motorcycle which creates a wind-chill factor of Arctic intensity. Well, modern technology is an amazing thing. On days when it is a little chilly, I wear properly layered modern fabrics, and I turn on the heated handgrips and heated seat on the motorcycle. But when it gets really cold, I don my heated jacket, heated gloves, and heated socks—which all plug into the motorcycle! And I ride along, in subfreezing temperatures, warm as toast. My point is, there may be a reasonable way to deal with some of the restrictions.

Exercise

It needs to happen every day. Or as close to every day as possible. Which means it gobbles up at least an hour of every day.

Excessive physical exercise

This is the limitation of not being able to "overdo it"— and that means in either the aerobic sense of exercising too long, or in the physical sense of lifting things too heavy. I think the real risk here is the inadvertent exceeding of the limits. For instance, it's easy to walk out the door, see two inches of snow, and start to clear your front steps—it's equally as easy to continue down your front sidewalk, up and down your driveway, and then help the neighbors. What might be okay for three minutes, clearing the steps, could unintentionally become excessive. Same with lifting heavy objects, don't get carried away.

Travel

A couple things here. Now, when I travel I always take a set of "backup pills"—this is a bottle that contains enough of my critical medications to cover me in case my other meds get lost. I give this bottle to my traveling companion, so it won't get lost with my own pills. (If I am traveling alone, the backup pills go in my pants pocket and are never separated from me.)

If I am traveling overseas, I also take a copy of every one of my prescriptions. In the United States, I am not worried about refilling prescriptions should they get lost, but what happens overseas? I'm not taking any chances.

Also, if traveling overseas I purchase an additional insurance policy that will cover any necessary hospital stay, and will cover medical transportation back to the US. These policies are not expensive and, for someone who has a higher likelihood of having a medical problem that most, can provide a much better level of coverage should anything go wrong.

Where's the hospital?

In the early years, immediately following my heart attack, I worried about being on an airplane. After all, what would happen if I had a heart attack while flying, with no access to a hospital? At some point, I realized I just had to get over this fear—otherwise I would never be able to be on a plane, boat, or in any situation that had me worrying about hospital access.

It initially disturbed me that there were any limitations at all, but I have learned to live with them, and not be resentful or bitter. There are a few things that take time—exercise, appointments, etc., but these things have not taken over my life. And there are a few limitations, but in many cases I have found "workarounds". For me, living with heart disease has really been about "beating" heart disease—staying alive. The tough part has been figuring out what needs to be changed, because even the best doctors can't tell you exactly what is going to work for you—the easier part has been making, and living, the changes.

Food

When I was in the hospital I was on a "low sodium, low cholesterol, low fat, no sugar, no caffeine diet"; it was horrible. For dinner they would bring me things like decaf tea, a dinner plate with a piece of boiled skinless plain white meat chicken and some steamed beans, a salad of lettuce and tomato no dressing, and a pear. Well, I am here to tell you that you actually can eat a healthy diet, and it doesn't have to consist of plain boiled skinless chicken; it can be tasty and satisfying.

If you have the kind of heart disease I do, atherosclerosis ("hardening of the arteries", "narrowing of the arteries", etc.), then you need to keep your cholesterol low. You also need to keep your blood pressure from becoming too high, and your heartbeat steady. So you need to take medications, exercise, and eat properly.

But why do you need to eat properly, especially when statins are so good that they can lower your cholesterol dramatically? There are several reasons:

- ♥ As effective as statins are at lowering your cholesterol, those results will only be improved by eating properly. Don't settle for an "OK" cholesterol level when you can have an outstanding level.
- ♥ Though statins may lower your cholesterol they will do nothing to help control your weight. We know over-weight and heart disease go hand-in-hand, and the most effective way to combat this is through healthy eating, and exercise.
- ♥ As good as statins are . . . and I've been told by cardiologists that statins are really great and have dramatically impacted the frequency and extent of heart attacks . . . as good as statins are, *an appropriate weight loss is 10 times more effective!*

108

Shortly after my heart attack, my friend Colleen advised, "Focus on the door opening, not the door closing." Great advice, and I say to you—focus on the foods you can eat, not the foods you can't.

Likely you've been told to eat foods low in cholesterol and fat, and low in sodium. You've also likely been told that sugar is not really great for you.

Right from the beginning I recognized how lucky I was to actually like certain foods. Turkey, I love turkey—so that opens the world of turkey subs and sandwiches, turkey for dinner, turkey burgers on the grill. Pasta, I love pasta—and it can be just a bowl of pasta with a little bit of olive oil and a sprinkling of parmesan cheese.

I have found things, and created things, that taste good, and are low in sodium, fat, cholesterol and sugar. The key is finding acceptable foods, which you like, so you don't feel like you are denying yourself the foods you want.

When I eat at home, I have a very consistent menu. Below is a sample weekly menu—which really isn't a sample, it is *my* weekly menu, and I vary from it rarely:

Breakfast, the same *every* day:
    ½ cup oatmeal, with skim milk & raisins (or blueberries)
Lunch, the same *every* day:
    "Skinny Elvis" (see recipe in Appendix)
Dinner *every* Monday & Tuesday:
    Homemade chili, or homemade gumbo, or homemade
    jambalaya (see recipes)
Dinner *every* Wednesday & Thursday:
    Pasta and broccoli in olive oil, with garlic
Dinner *every* Friday:
    Asian noodle soup dinner, usually Vietnamese
Dinner *every* Saturday:
    Broiled salmon, asparagus, sweet potato
Dinner *every* Sunday:
    Turkey burger, corn on the cob, kale salad

And I guess what surprises people is—this is what I eat, *year round*. I can't tell you how many times I've heard, "Don't you get tired of eating the same things?" Well, no. It's all things that I like, and don't tire of. The bowl of oatmeal tastes good and fills me until lunch. The Skinny Elvis, with its peanut butter, honey and banana flavors is delicious and filling. There is enough variety in my dinners that I look forward to them each week. And my late night snacks are all low-fat low-cholesterol.

We eat out sometimes, and when we do, I just make certain to eat meals that conform to my needs. If it's lunchtime I get a turkey sandwich with lettuce and tomato (no mayo). If it's dinner I nearly always get some kind of fish, grilled or broiled—and never with butter or a cream sauce. Or I find pasta with seafood or shellfish made in olive oil (no butter).

There is enough variety, and enough flavor, that I have no difficulty staying away from the sugary, salty, fried or fatty foods that clogged my arteries.

So what diet should you follow? You'll notice I've avoided the word "diet" throughout this book, because it is not about sticking to a diet; it is about making healthy choices. If I were you, I would stay away from all the fad diets and published diets; they are restrictive by nature, which is why people eventually "cheat" and ultimately fail.

You don't need to be restricted by "a diet". The world of food is still open to you—you just need to make healthy choices for your ingredients and your meals.

Eating "low-everything" food isn't as bad as it sounds.
I have found new foods that I absolutely love.

The "Mississippi River Delta"

New Orleans lies on the banks of the Mighty Mississippi River to the north of the Mississippi River Delta. Many times over the years we spent a "long weekend", four or five days, enjoying the music, the history, and, of course, the food in New Orleans. So many times in fact that we had a routine—favorite restaurants, favorite spots to listen to music, favorite walks. We enjoyed it so much, we decided to plan a longer visit.

Trouble was, when I started to calculate the cost for a hotel for, say, 10 days, it was enormous. A nice hotel in the French Quarter, eating out three meals a day—we're talking a small fortune for just the hotel, not to mention the meals.

Which led me to start looking for rentals, and led me to Cile and Gregg. About my age, Gregg moved to New Orleans as a young man, to play for the New Orleans Saints. When injury ended his professional football career he pursued his passion for physical fitness and opened a health club. Cile, who was his business partner, is my vision of a modern southern belle—beautiful, educated, well-spoken, sophisticated. Sadly, Hurricane Katrina destroyed their health clubs, but fortunately it did not destroy their home on the other side of Lake Pontchartrain, or their beautiful 1790s house in the French Quarter, which they were kind enough to rent to us for a month.

Furnished in period décor from the 1800s, with a circular staircase, a private courtyard, and a balcony overlooking Bourbon Street, the home is equipped with all the modern amenities. Three beautiful bathrooms, flat screen TVs, Wi-Fi *and* a full modern kitchen! Which gives me terrific flexibility with food.

I decided (and notice I said *I decided*, because a decision that involves what I eat is mine, mine alone, and I neither intend to impose the decision on others nor cave to others' eating plans), I decided that I would stock the kitchen with all the things needed to maintain my daily breakfast and lunch menu, exactly as I eat at home. And if you review my weekly menu, it's pretty simple, as I eat exactly the same breakfast and lunch daily; the only thing I had to do was ship a supply of Reduced Fat Peanut Butter ahead of time.

And I decided that I would go out to dinner every night. Not only go out every night, but make an overt attempt to explore many more of the great New Orleans restaurants than just our few favorites. A bit challenging—"New Orleans' 300 Essential Restaurants" was my starting point (there are roughly 1,500 restaurants in New Orleans! And as far as I can tell, there is not one single national chain restaurant in the French Quarter.)

A few points about my menu plan:

♥ First: It wasn't just Rashmika and I on this trip. Having rented a house we invited friends and family, so at various times we had one, two or three guests staying with us. How was I going to maintain my breakfast and lunch discipline without being rude?

♥ Second: Eating out 30 nights in a row! How was I going to do this without overloading on rich, or fatty, foods? Or just foods my system was unaccustomed to dealing with?

♥ Third: Eating two meals home and one out every day is much less expensive than eating out every meal. Can you imagine the cost of 90 meals in restaurants in one month? (Or another way to think of it—can you imagine how much I saved by eating 60 meals at home?)

Cile and Gregg's place is in a terrific central location, right in the middle of the French Quarter. Fifty feet from Bourbon Street, a block from Jackson Square, a block from Preservation Hall, two blocks from Café Du Monde. Such a great location that, like on all our prior trips to the French Quarter, we made no plan to rent a car. We could walk everywhere, but on the rare occasions that we wanted to leave the French Quarter we could take a cab. And, when I told Cile and Gregg our plans, they actually left bicycles at the house for us!

So about a half hour after we arrived, we trekked over to Rouse's Market, a block away, and carried back the staples we needed. Bread, honey, skim milk, oatmeal, raisins, bottled water, popcorn, frozen yogurt, bananas. So now I was set for breakfast and lunch!

I stuck to the plan; every morning while my oatmeal was cooling I walked briskly over to either Community Coffee or Café Du Monde and got a large steaming cup of chicory coffee or Café Americana for Rashmika. When we had guests, either we all ate breakfast at home or we went to the Camellia Grill, which was a blast—they only offer counter service (no tables), the staff is outgoing and gregarious and is dressed in starched white chefs' outfits, and they have a traditional breakfast menu. The food is great, the staff is fun, and the price is right . . . which is probably why they've been around since the 1940s. Actually, the place has a 40s feel. And I had no trouble ordering from their traditional menu; this was not a repeat of my 1980s New Orleans breakfast episode!

Lunches, also stuck to the plan. On most days I would walk over to Chef Paul Prudhomme's restaurant, K-Paul's Louisiana Kitchen, and take out one of their great salads for Rashmika, then make my normal "Skinny Elvis". When guests came and we decided to eat lunch out, we either selected a place where I knew I could get an "acceptable" lunch (like a grilled chicken salad), or I ate my Skinny Elvis before we left, and enjoyed a cup or two of decaf cappuccino and conversation while everyone else ate their lunch.

Dinner, this was a little more interesting, but I also stuck to the plan. My original idea was "30 restaurants in 30 days" for dinner. I hadn't initially considered how much I like Commander's Palace, which is far and away the finest in New Orleans, perhaps the finest in the country. So months before the trip we made 4 reservations for Commander's, one a week, which incidentally included Thanksgiving dinner. I also hadn't initially anticipated that we would stumble on a place, like K-Paul's, that we would like so much that we would be compelled to repeat. As it worked out, we did eat out all 30 nights, in 15 different restaurants.

But in every one of those 15 restaurants I ate Cajun, or creole, or regional food—I did not limit myself to only those foods I eat at home, or only those spices I am accustomed to. I tried to eat real New Orleans food, so I asked about gumbo at every restaurant (there's as many kinds of gumbo as there are restaurants!); if they had gumbo I got a small bowl or a cup to start each dinner. I looked for fish on the menus; then I told them that I was unable to eat anything made with cream or butter. I had some of the best fish, vegetables and combinations you could imagine.

One Saturday afternoon I received a call from Commander's Palace, apologizing to me that our "regular table" (hmm, I didn't know we had a regular table) would not be available the following evening, but they would be seating us at The Reagan Table. "The Reagan table?" I asked—realizing I hadn't pronounced all the capital letters they did—and they explained that this was Ron and Nancy's favorite table. I certainly felt honored they thought that highly of us!

So the next evening after we were seated in the elegant circular corner location overlooking the main dining room, I noticed a delicious sounding fish entrée on the menu. Of course, it looked like something that would have to be smothered in butter to give it the rich flavor described on the menu, so I inquired as to whether they could make it for me, sans any butter or cream.

The staff returned with our meals a short time later. As is the tradition at Commander's there was enough staff to place everyone's plate in front of them at the same instant. It all looked delicious. I took my first bite of the fish, and it was absolutely wonderful . . . so wonderful in fact that I knew they got my order confused, and made it with butter by mistake. I signaled the waitress, explained the situation, and she hustled off, my plate in hand.

She returned perhaps 90 seconds later, plate in hand. I was thinking, "How the heck could they re-make this so fast?" "Mr. Segal," she said, "Chef Tory wants to assure you there is absolutely no butter, lard, cream or anything like that in your meal. He says he would never put butter in your food." I was stunned. First, I just can't tell you how indescribably good this food was; impossible to imagine someone preparing something this tasty, this rich, this smooth, without butter! And second, that Commander's actually knew how to cook for me. I asked the waiter to extend both my apology and my gratitude to Chef Tory . . . and went on to enjoy one of the best meals of my life!

The experience at Commander's was outstanding, but to a lesser degree I experienced similar results elsewhere. Wherever we went for dinner my request was the same—no butter, no cream. There seems to be a pride amongst restaurants and chefs in New Orleans that I have rarely experienced elsewhere; they want to cook you a great meal, and are actually proud to showcase their skill in being able to do that even in circumstances like mine, where they are not permitted to use some of their most effective culinary ingredients.

Thirty great dinners! All with savory tastes and smells like nothing I'd had before. All prepared with no butter, no cream. It is doable; you don't have to be limited to a piece of skinless white chicken and lettuce!

About halfway through our stay I realized I really needed Cajun and creole food at home. I spent a couple days at the New Orleans School of Cooking in the French Quarter. The classes are inexpensive and fun, and I have since then adapted some of their recipes with heart-healthy ingredients. I have included some of these in the recipes that appear in the Appendix.

Oh, and the Mississippi Delta? So we spent a month in New Orleans. I stuck to my eating plan for breakfasts and lunches, and had 30 amazing dinners at great restaurants. And Rashmika was pretty good about her eating . . . at least initially. Let me mention, she has no health issues that require special foods or preparation.

She started the month with strict portion control, dividing her plate into what would be eaten, and what would not; most obvious were the desserts, which she cut in half. I noticed as the month went on the portion of uneaten dessert kept shrinking; by the end, the uneaten portion was one spoonful!

For that month we both walked or bicycled everywhere, so we should have been burning off more calories than in our normal lives, where we always seem to hop into a car to go anywhere.

Nonetheless, a few days prior to leaving New Orleans I started thinking that I would really have to watch what I eat for a while after I got home, as surely the 30 great dinners in a row added unwanted pounds.

A few days after I got home I stepped on the scale . . SURPRISE! . . I lost 11 pounds! I dropped from 173 to 162! And the Mississippi Delta? That would be 33 pounds, the difference between what I lost, and what Rashmika gained.

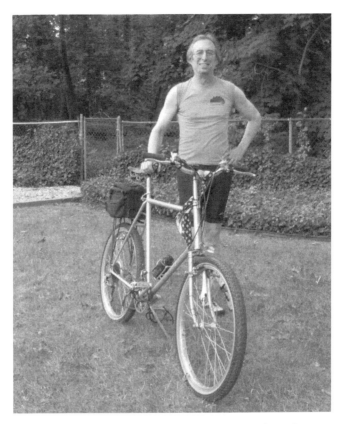

"Twenty-six years after the heart attack . . ."
(P.S. Same bike, same shirt, different glasses.)

Maybe My Life's Not Ruined!

Twenty-six years after the heart attack I realize I have lived a great life, in spite of the heart attack; in spite of the limitations and the necessities. Or is it because of the heart attack?

Because it made me value my precious time here? Because it made me focus on the aspects of life that are truly important, truly valuable? Like using the time I have wisely, doing what was important to me, rather than what was required or expected by others.

Like retiring when I was 51 years old. Many people mistakenly think I'm a wealthy man, and that I was simply able to walk away from work. Nope—but two significant events compelled my decision for an early retirement.

The first was the death of my father, who dreamt of retiring to Florida someday. In the summertime he wore powder blue slacks, white leather shoes and a white leather belt . . . just like the old men in Florida. Unfortunately colon cancer took him when he was 59 years old, before he ever had the chance to retire. I didn't want to suffer the same fate as my father.

The second reason you already know: "We will see." I can die . . . today, tomorrow, anytime.

When I realized I might live, I resolved to retire as young as possible. By the time I was 45, I was thinking about how to do it. I did not have a requirement to have a huge nest egg; my goal was that I simply could make ends meet. Because what I was looking for from retirement was not a lavish life of jetting around the world, of five star restaurants or of beaches in the Caribbean. What I was looking for was liberation from the agenda of others, to have control of my own time.

So at 51, I semi-retired, having projected that I would have nearly enough to get by, and taking a leap of faith that I would be able to develop some other small sources of revenue (buying and selling motorcycle and drum parts on eBay, consulting, and authoring, designing and publishing music education books)—and the result is, so far, 12 years of pursuing my own agenda. And I wouldn't trade those 12 years for the big bank account I may have had, because I realize that more precious than money is my time, and my health.

I have lived a great life, seeing our children grow, doing amazing things with my time, and accomplishing things professionally I never even dreamt of. For several years after the heart attack, I really thought my life would be cut short by heart disease, but I've had ten thousand days since then.

You can do a lot in ten thousand days. Even if you have to spend time exercising, going to doctor appointments and taking pills.

I didn't believe I would be able to live a full or satisfying life; I thought my activities would be so restricted as to leave me unfulfilled. But here I am, age 63, juggling, drumming, riding bicycles and motorcycles, writing, traveling . . . . and eating fat free frozen yogurt, Skinny Elvises and air-popped popcorn.

Let me tell you what the universe has shown me in ten thousand days . . . and I'll put it in three buckets, first are the great things that happen in most people's lives (provided they live long enough), second are amazing things I did or participated in, and third are professional accomplishments.

Family—the moments we all live for:

Almost exactly a year after the heart attack, I gazed up to the stars on a crystal clear summer night, and took in the crisp ocean air, thankful to be alive. I was in a grandstand just off the boardwalk in Atlantic City, with Stephen and Samantha on either side of me. I got to take my children, ages 13 and 11, to their first rock concert, the Beach Boys on the Fourth of July!

A few years later, Kathy and I divorced, opening new worlds to us both. We managed throughout to maintain good relationships with our children and with each other. We danced and cried at the weddings of our children years later; once again, Kathy is joining us to celebrate Thanksgiving later this year.

Later, I met and married Rashmika. We've had almost 8,000 days together, all post-heart attack. She's only ever known me as a person who refuses to smoke or eat dessert. We've enjoyed a twenty year relationship, which seems to get better over the years.

I've seen our children grow into amazing adults. We danced at their weddings and cried at the birth of our grand-daughter. After admiring the way Stephen pursued his life dream of being a writer and editor, I was seated with the dignitaries at the Palais des Congrès in Montreal the night he was honored with a Hugo Award (the "Oscar" of the worlds of science fiction and fantasy). Following an average high school career, we watched Samantha blossom in college, completing a degree in psychology, and going on to law school (I actually got to administer her oath of office in New Jersey!); I was stunned, shocked, six years later when she was made New York City's youngest administrative law judge, at just 29 years old! And our daughter-in-law Stacy, who we've known since college, has made us so proud by following her dream to protect and defend mistreated animals; she has worked tirelessly, traveling the country, living away from home for months on end, to defend and rescue mistreated horses wherever they are. Now with the ASCPA in New York City, she has become one of the most prominent equine cruelty specialists in the world.

Seven years after the heart attack I brought home Genghis, a 7-week-old Shar-Pei puppy; he loved Rashmika and I and Samantha, hated everyone else! Eight years later when Genghis died too young, we adopted Vito, a 140-pound bullmastiff; the fiercest looking dog you could imagine, Vito loved just everyone! He became a certified therapy dog, and took me on weekly visits to terminal patients at the Barbara E. Cheung Memorial Hospice, something I would have never even dreamt of doing without Vito.

I had the joy of holding our granddaughter in my arms the day after she was born, 22 years after my heart attack. Ever since, I've had the pleasure of watching Rashmika, who never raised children of her own and never really spent time with a child, discover the beauty and wonder of helping a child grow, learn and flourish.

And . . . I have actually survived long enough to be the oldest male in some branches of our family—my Hawaiian relatives tell me I am the family's kupuna!

Some things I've done that still amaze me:

While I haven't done anything of the magnitude of a Charles Lindbergh or a Malcolm Forbes or Rollie Free, considering at one time I never expected to live anything more than a life of declining health, I have done, and continue to do, things that amaze and delight me.

I was blown away when, just six months after the heart attack, I found myself listening to real, live Dixieland jazz at Preservation Hall just off Bourbon Street! I imagined how it was when Louis Armstrong played the same songs in the same clubs, how it was when Al Jolson wandered into a similar New Orleans jazz club, and started down the path that led to stardom. I was so taken with the music, the food, the culture, the history, that we return to New Orleans regularly. For years we went annually for a "long weekend"; now we try to stay for a month, immersing ourselves in the sights, sounds, smells and tastes of the French Quarter. And it just keeps getting better!

Every year Stephen and I go on a week-long father-son vacation . . . to the World Science Fiction Convention. We have traveled to three continents and made many friends. One year we sat for an hour, alone with George Takei, and discussed inequality and prejudice. One year we listened to Ray Bradbury, 86 years old, reminisce about his childhood and his early days as a struggling author. I coordinate an annual event called "Stroll With The Stars"; I lure people out for a healthy morning walk by bringing along great authors, artists and editors. (Close to 500 people showed up for the four strolls in Chicago last year!) We have strolled through the streets of Montreal, Yokohama, Glasgow, Chicago, Denver with Boris Vallejo, Connie Willis, John Scalzi, Larry Niven, Frank Wu and too many more to mention.

I can't even guess how much time I spent on motorcycles, but in '95 Rashmika and I rode 4,000 miles, from the East Coast to Devils Tower in Wyoming, and back across Canada. We saw the wonders of the Dakotas, the Badlands where Teddy Roosevelt sought isolation in the despair following the death of his young wife and his mother, the majestic Crazy Horse Memorial, an immense mountain carving that dwarfs Mount Rushmore and is the living dream of sculptor Korczak, whose family carries on the carving daily, 65 years after he began, and 31 years after his death. It was a trip few would imagine a person with heart disease could make. When I was 50 years old Tom and I rode Screamin' Eagle Harley-Davidsons from New Jersey to North Carolina and back . . . in one day . . . leaving at 6 a.m. and riding continuously, except for gas stops, until midnight. 1,010 miles in 18 hours, earning us memberships in the Iron Butt Association, "The World's Toughest Riders".

We've seen amazing concerts and shows, over 120 so far. Everyone from Bob Dylan and Paul Simon . . . to "South Pacific" and "Phantom of the Opera" . . . to Dixieland jazz in smoky clubs and military bands in front of Edinburgh Castle . . . and tons of other great performers. I regretted not seeing the Beatles in the 60s, but I did see Paul McCartney in 1990, and Ringo in 2011. Luckily, but sadly, we saw Peter, Paul and Mary in their final performance before the passing of Mary Travers. We also stumbled into a blues club one night in New Orleans, and caught Eric Burdon performing "House of the Rising Sun"—talk about being in the right place at the right time!

We've eaten some memorable meals, something that may sound odd coming from a person who maintains very strict discipline about what he eats. Commander's Palace in New Orleans, perhaps the finest restaurant in the US, where they prepare the most delicious meals you could imagine (and, within my dietary guidelines!) and treat you like an old friend every time you walk in the door. The Russian Tea Room, where they seated Christian

Slater next to us. Peter Luger[4] in Brooklyn, one of the worlds' great steakhouses, indescribable with its brusque waiters and incomparable steaks. Again, remember: I am not in that top one-percent who have money to burn, I'm just a guy who wants to experience what the world has to offer, and I'm not shy about making reservations at nice places!

I learned to juggle knives, at age 55. I had been juggling since I was about 35, but I would occasionally see someone juggle knives, or fire, and think, "Why not me?" (Except for the obvious—fingers, toes, pain!) Knowing how people would react, I practiced this for a year in privacy. One day while practicing I looked up, and realized Rashmika had found me out; her comment might have been, um, scathing; for the record, I have not yet lost any fingers or toes. And before you ask about chainsaws, think about how hard it is to juggle 20-inch double-edged knives.

Rashmika and I are huge fans of Ferrari; we love seeing the bright red cars with the Prancing Horse blistering around the racetracks of the world. In '09 we actually sat in the hairpin turn in Montreal and watched them fight for the win in the Grand Prix du Canada. In 2012 my friend Rick called, and said "You won't believe it, Groupon has a deal to drive Ferraris and Lamborghinis on a racetrack . . . for 100 bucks!" Seemed too good to be true, but it wasn't—Rick, Rashmika and I all got to actually drive Ferraris on a racetrack. Foot to the floor in a Ferrari F430, with a 500 horsepower engine screaming right behind your head, is a genuine thrill. Given my "carpe diem" attitude, I really did get to see how fast a Ferrari goes!

About five years ago I put two four-by-four "square foot gardens" in our yard, and in '07 we tasted our first crop of homegrown peppers. Now we flavor all our chili, jambalaya and gumbo with homegrown habaneros, chilis, Italian long hots and Indian tejaswini peppers.

---

[4] OK, I'll admit that at Peter Luger it's a little tough to order a low-cholesterol meal. However, I visit Peter Luger every 10th year, on my 50th birthday, my 60th birthday, etc. This is the only time I eat steak; I would consider a 10 year interval "moderation".

At 60 years old, 23 years after the heart attack, I started to regret that I gave up the study of drumming in my early teens. I found a brilliant drummer and music teacher, Jimmy Sica, who started by teaching me to read music. Since then he and I have become fast friends; in 2012 we published our first book, "How To Read Drum Music". It is heartwarming to us both to see the monthly sales figures, and know that people in the US, the UK and Europe are learning to read music from our book.

And then there was work:

I spent 24 years in a banking career—15 years before the heart attack and nine after. And then I moved into a second career, in the motorcycle business.

I did many things in banking, but over the years people started referring to me as an ATM expert, or an "ATM guru" (of course I knew this wasn't true, having spent time with the true visionaries and gurus). About five years after the heart attack I was stunned when I was appointed to a seat on the Board of Directors of the New York Cash Exchange, at the time the largest ATM network in the US, and started participating in the decisions which shaped our industry.

Though some of my work on ATMs still impacts the way people do business with their bank cards today, I can you tell the greatest accomplishment from my banking career has emerged in recent years, watching the development of some of the people who were on my team over the years. Many of them have developed into wonderful family people and pillars of their communities, and some have gone on to be senior managers, even presidents, of companies.

Ten years after the heart attack, my friend Tom and I opened Liberty Harley-Davidson, in Rahway, New Jersey, where Harley had closed down their original dealership a few years earlier. The customer base felt abandoned, and was angry. We worked diligently to win the customers' confidence, and year later we were honored as one of the "Top 100 Dealerships" in the United States. I sold my interest to Tom in 2001, and he and his family have built the dealership into the premiere Harley franchise in the New York metro area, winning accolades year after year.

Harley-Davidson Motorcycle Company drafted me to be on the Advisory Board of H-D Financial Services, which provides loans to both their customers and their dealers, and I once again found myself helping make decisions which affected an entire industry.

In 2004 my friends Dan and Ray and I, along with seven other friends (including Tom), opened the largest Honda dealership east of the Mississippi. Since then we have expanded the dealership to three buildings, selling motorcycles, ATVs, jetskis, dirtbikes and power equipment from BMW, CanAm, Ducati, Honda, Husqvarna, Kawasaki, Piaggio, Polaris, SeaDoo, Triumph, Vespa and Victory. This dealership has also been honored as one of the "Top 100" in the US, and was voted "The Best Motorcycle Dealership in Central Jersey" in the annual customer poll.

Since 1998 we have made 15,000 people smile by putting them on the motorcycle of their dreams—*15,000!* Men, women, children—some on big bikes to tour the country, some on dirtbikes or ATVs to ride with their friends, some on jetskis to enjoy the Jersey shore. Some of the most passionate have been the new Harley owners; many thanked me, but a few were so happy that they hugged me, or shook my hand, with tears in their eyes. More than one told me this was "the best day of his life".

When Hurricane Sandy devastated New Jersey in 2012, leaving families without power or heat for days or weeks on end, my partners and our employees stepped up . . . opening the dealership, which incidentally also had no power, at 6 a.m. each day and working until midnight. Everyone chipping in. We were able to provide prepped, running, gassed up generators to 800 families! We even had some employees who, after leaving work at midnight, went to homes of the elderly or infirmed, set up generators, and taught the folks how to operate them. I have never been prouder of anything in my professional life than I was of the way our business responded in this time of need.

Don't assume, or plan, to die young.
Do the things that make your life complete,
but don't do things that will shorten it.

Are there things I haven't done as a result of my heart condition? Sure. But given the ten thousand days I've lived, and the things I have done, do the omissions really matter? So I can't eat Black Forest Cake or Boston Cream Pie—I can't lie in the sun baking on the beach—I can't stay outdoors for hours and shovel snow. While I may have liked doing some of these things, I certainly don't regret avoiding them to extend my life.

I have lived, and continue to live, a very full life—something I never thought would happen. I've been lucky; but I've also proactively and continuously managed my health. I hope you have some luck like I have, and make the most of it.

Afterword
by Dr. Ian J. Molk

Writing an afterword about the cardiac journey of my patient, Stu Segal, is challenging. Challenging in the sense that it is hard to do justice to the rather remarkable makeover Stu has managed to achieve.

Stu's passion and appreciation of life is very evident in his narrative. His experience has taught him that good health is by far the most important possession in life. He has realized that it is the most essential ingredient in much sought after formula of an enjoyable and fulfilling life.

There is a dictum that I use constantly with many patients: "You cannot take your health for granted—you have to pay attention to it and work at it. It is the most important work that you can do." Stu has embraced this dictum with a vigor that is rare. He is an outstanding example of someone who has taken the bull by the horns and made dramatic changes with admirable results.

He carries with him a sense of humility and appreciation of life that dovetails with another dictum that I frequently use: "Health is not an entitlement. You have to earn it!" Stu has earned it.

It has been a privilege and a pleasure to have been Stu's cardiologist for the past 20 years or so. He has done a truly commendable job in turning his health around for the better. He is the type of patient that makes practicing cardiology enormously rewarding and satisfying.

Hopefully this book will motivate many victims of coronary artery disease to take control of their own destiny and do the work that will greatly improve their quality of life and prognosis. Stu has.

Afterword
by Stu Segal

In the summer of '09 at the World Science Fiction Convention in Montreal I met a young man named Neil Clarke, the publisher/editor of *Clarkesworld Magazine*, an online science fiction and fantasy magazine.

Neil was especially busy at that convention, championing an effort to keep an entire category of magazines eligible for award recognition. He had worked for months leading up to that convention, in fact, mobilizing fans from around the world.

A couple years later, on the way home from another Worldcon, Neil and I were stuck in the Houston airport waiting for thunderstorms over New York to clear. Through our six hours of kibitzing in the airport I learned that Neil is a family man, a loving father and husband. I learned that in addition to spending full time working on *Clarkesworld*, he was a full time employee of a local private school.

My feeling after six hours one on one: Neil struck me as the cream of the crop. Much like my own son, friendly, talented, articulate, hard-working, loving—a real credit to the world of science fiction and fantasy.

In the summer of 2012, word spread like wildfire across the blogosphere that Neil, while attending a convention in Boston, had suffered a heart attack. People were shocked, because much like me when I had a heart attack, Neil was young, and outwardly a picture of health and fitness—trim and active, certainly not the person you'd expect to be stricken. Well luckily, but also scarily, his family was there with him on vacation, and could be there with him for an extra week and a half as he stabilized in the hospital and was eventually released.

When I heard of Neil's situation it threw me back 25 years; for the first time in decades I thought about my own experience, having a heart attack, young, out of the blue. How difficult it was to accept. How challenging it was to adjust. I wanted desperately to come up with some words of wisdom to help Neil through the crisis and into the future.

I called Neil a few weeks later and could tell he was in the same place I had been. Fighting hard to accept the situation and make the best of it. As time unfolded, Neil had to deal with some of the same issues I did; but he also had to deal with a somewhat different diagnosis than I had, resulting in the implant of a defibrillator (not so common for a 45-year-old), and some other non-heart related medical issues.

After my conversation with Neil I tried to find him some information—a book, a website—that talked to his situation. I couldn't find it. I couldn't really find anything written for young victims of unexpected heart attacks. Which led me to write this book—for people like Neil. It is my hope this book will help someone cope—will help someone realize that a heart attack doesn't necessarily have to be the end of their life; it could well be a beginning.

And by the way, fourteen months after the heart attack, Neil won his third Hugo Award.

appendix

Top Ten for a Healthy Heart

10. Stay educated about new developments in heart treatment.[5]

9. One glass of wine a day.[6]

8. Avoid depression. Learn its symptoms and confront them —
with help if need be.

7. Learn not to get stressed.

6. Keep your weight under control.

5. Exercise every day. Or as close to every day as possible.

4. No smoking. Ever.

3. Stick to doing what you know you should — don't be swayed by
peer pressure. Cheating, even at the "holiday season", will only
hurt one person — you.

2. Take your meds, faithfully, on time.

1. Enjoy life. A happy person is more likely to be a healthy person.

---

[5] A good resource is the monthly "Harvard Heart Letter", written for patients. See
http://www.health.harvard.edu/newsletters/Harvard_Heart_Letter
[6] One glass of wine a day, unless your physician recommends otherwise.

Lessons Learned

These are in no particular order. (You'll recognize some from preceding chapters.)

I can die. Today, tomorrow, anytime.

Clogged arteries can kill me. I can't control my genes, but I can control my eating, exercise, smoking and stress.

Life is not always fair.

Never change a winning game. Always change a losing game.

RELAX! Most upsetting things are really not "life and death", and are not worth getting stressed.

Depression only makes everything worse. Learn its symptoms and confront them—with help if need be. If depression begins, deal with it immediately.

Don't smoke the "next" cigarette. Don't eat the next dessert.

I still hate exercise, but admit that it actually makes me feel better. And it helps keep me alive.

I need to take my meds. Consistently—every day, same time.

Thin=Healthy: Not necessarily true. (But being overweight is definitely a problem for a heart patient.)

A heart condition is not going to stop me from living my life. There is a way.

Doctors are very cautious and they don't always understand my priorities.

It's not about the Destination, it's about the Journey.

Do the things that make my life complete. Do them now.

Find the best doctors I can, but accept that I need to manage my own health, no one else can. Not my doctor, not my therapist, not my spouse. Me.

There are foods that taste just as good as a burger and fries, that won't clog my arteries.

I can change. I have willpower. The changes I need are for me, no one else.

Eating "low-everything" food isn't as bad as it sounds. I have found new foods that I absolutely love.

I can't assume, or plan, to die young. I must do the things that make my life complete, but not the things that will cut it short.

Stop assuming the way things are is the way they should be. Focus on what is important; ignore the unimportant.

Heart-Healthy Recipes

I have included some recipes that work for me—including my Health Chili (low fat, low sodium), which actually won 3rd place in an open chili cook-off against 30 other contestants with their traditional artery-clogging entries. I am very proud of this because it was based on the popular votes of several hundred people who all tasted the various chilis, had no idea mine was made with healthful ingredients, and nonetheless voted it 3rd out of 30, proving my point that you can indeed make heart-healthy food that tastes just as good as artery-clogging food.

Over the years I have developed a few recipes around these criteria:

- ♥ Tastes good
- ♥ Good for me (or, at least, not bad)
- ♥ Easy to make

While some of the recipes have a lot of ingredients, you will notice they are all cooked the easy way, in a Crock-Pot. There may be some chopping, but ultimately it all gets thrown in the pot, you go about your business and at the end of the day, voila!, cooked to perfection.

I also try to cook in large enough quantities that the majority can be frozen, and easily defrosted for future meals. The Crock-Pot is perfect as it lets me cook enough for weeks in advance.

"Skinny Elvis"

You've probably heard of Elvis Presley's legendary lunches of fried peanut butter and banana sandwiches, sometimes with honey, other times with bacon. Always grilled in a quarter pound of butter, grilled until all the butter is absorbed by the sandwich (talk about a heart-stopper special!)

Here's a tasty variation that has enough substance to get you through the day. I eat this for lunch every day, have for the last 10 years, and it still tastes great to me!

This is what you need:
    Wheat bread
    A banana
    Honey
    Reduced fat peanut butter

Drizzle some honey on 2 pieces of wheat bread. Spread reduced-fat peanut butter over the honey. Slice a banana and put it between the two pieces of bread.

Now heat up a small frying pan, spray it with butter flavored cooking spray, and grill the sandwich until the bread is somewhat toasted. (Note the cooking spray has 0 fat, 0 cholesterol and 0 sodium.)

Truth is, I rarely ever grill the Skinny Elvis, I'm too lazy. Instead I just toast the bread first, drip on the honey while the toast is still warm, and make the sandwich. Takes maybe 3 minutes to make. It's perfect with a glass of skim milk.

Chili

The goal here is to have a tasty, filling chili, that's not loaded with fat or sodium. And it needs to taste like real chili.

(BTW: I tried to come up with a clever name for this recipe. Heart Healthy Chili? Sweet Potato Gobbler Chili? I am open to any suggestions for an appropriate name.)

The way to accomplish this is to use lowfat meat and tasty ingredients. Also note, this gets cooked in a Crock-Pot, which means you prepare the ingredients, throw them in the pot, and let them cook—so you also get the benefit of the aroma all day while it cooks!

This is what you need:

16 oz. tomato sauce
32 oz. beer (light beer, not dark)
¾ tbsp. chili powder
2 tbsp. sugar
3/8 tsp. cayenne
1¼ tbsp. cumin
1 tbsp. paprika
2 squirts of hot sauce
2 tbsp. garlic
2 lbs. ground turkey
2 lbs. sweet potatoes

1 bag broccoli slaw
1 sweet red onion
1 yellow bell pepper
1 green bell pepper
1 red bell pepper
1 cooked ear of corn
30 oz. beans (pinto beans, red beans, black beans, or a combination)
3 tbsp. cornstarch,

1 Italian longhot pepper (optional)
1 cayenne pepper (optional)

Brown the ground turkey in a frying pan.
Cut the sweet potatoes into 1" square chunks.
Chop up the peppers and the onion.
Slice the kernels off the corn.

Put the beer and the tomato sauce in the Crock-Pot with the spices. Add everything except the beans and the cornstarch to the pot. The amount of hot peppers, or other spicy stuff, is up to you. Set the Crock-Pot on high for 1 hour, then low for 7 hours.

Add the beans and the cornstarch, and cook for 1 more hour on low.

I really like the taste of the sweet potatoes contrasting the spiciness of the peppers. But if you want a more traditional taste, use 4 lbs. of ground turkey instead of 2 lbs. turkey/2 lbs. sweet potatoes.

This will give you a really big pot of chili, which you can eat mixed 50/50 with rice. We use basmati rice, but you can use whatever rice you want. Also, you can put the chili in plastic containers, freeze it, and thaw it in the microwave when you want more. An easy dinner to make—thaw the chili, microwave some rice!

Seafood Chicken Andouille Gumbo

If you've ever been to New Orleans you know that one of the tastiest treats is the gumbo. There's all kinds of gumbo—Cajun, Creole, red, brown. They all have one thing in common, that unique New Orleans flavor that comes from a base of roux and "the trinity" (celery, onion, bell pepper). So our goal here is to achieve that unique flavor, without excess fat, no added salt and no butter.

This is what you need:

½ cup olive oil

½ cup flour

2 cups chopped onion

1 cup chopped bell pepper

½ cup chopped celery

4 cups seafood stock

2 cups diced tomatoes

2 lbs. boneless skinless chicken thighs, cut in pieces

1 lb. Andouille sausage

1 lb. frozen sliced okra

2 Indian peppers

1 Italian longhot pepper

Some minced garlic

1 tbsp. Joe's Stuff[7]

¾ tsp. cayenne pepper

Savoie's Light Roux

1 lb. shrimp (or 2 lbs.)

Cut the chicken and the sausage into pieces.

Make a roux in a sauté pan, using the flour and oil, or pick up some Savoie's Light Old Fashioned Roux. If you use Savoie's heat and thin with seafood stock, mixing until you get a flowing consistency. (I won't go into great detail on how to make a roux, but it is basically stirring the flour and fat constantly while it blends and cooks, until you get it to a the color and consistency of peanut butter. Being a heart patient, you can't use the traditional fat; use olive oil instead. It can be a tedious process; be careful, as olive oil burns easily, and if it burns you'll need to start over. Which is why I use Savoie's Light Roux.)

---

[7] Joe's Stuff is a blend of spices created by the New Orleans School of Cooking. A lot of folks have their own mixes of spices; I think the NOSC got it just right. Available at their website, www.neworleansschoolofcooking.com

When the roux is ready, add some a little seafood stock and the celery, onions and bell pepper. Cook for a short time, constantly stirring, just until the onions appear translucent.

Pour the roux/trinity mix into the Crock-Pot. Add the rest of the seafood stock, diced tomatoes, chicken, sausage, okra, some minced garlic, 1 tbsp. Joe's Stuff, ¾ tsp. cayenne pepper and some hot peppers (I use a couple Indian Tejaswini peppers and 1 Italian longhot pepper). Cook on low for 6 hours.

Add the shrimp. Cook for 1 hr. on high (or 1½ hour on low).

Serve the gumbo over white converted rice. (Heart patients note; I don't actually eat the Andouille sausage; I leave it for the non heart patients at the table. It is one of the essential flavors, but it pervades the dish, so you don't need to actually eat it to appreciate the flavor.)

Again, this is a dish that freezes well, and can be easily thawed and served over rice.

Creole Jambalaya

There's nothing quite like jambalaya . . . and yes, you can make a tasty low-sodium low-fat variation.

Even though this is made in the Crock-Pot like the chili and the gumbo, it won't yield as much—this is because the rice is included right in the recipe in the Crock-Pot. It also doesn't freeze quite as well as the others. That said, it's our favorite.

This is what you need:

2 tablespoons olive oil	2 hot peppers
2 cups chopped onion	2 14 oz., cans diced tomatoes
1 cup chopped bell pepper	1 lb. boneless skinless
1 cup chopped celery	chicken
3 cloves garlic, minced	1 lb. smoked sausage
1 tbsp. Joe's Stuff	2 cups converted rice
¾ tsp. cayenne pepper	1 lb. peeled medium shrimp
1½ cups seafood stock	¼ cup chopped parsley

Cut the chicken and the sausage into bite-sized pieces.

Heat the olive oil on high, and sauté the onion, celery and pepper stirring often, about 5 minutes, until the onions are translucent. Add the garlic and spices, stir and cook for 1 minute.

Remove from heat, add the seafood stock, stirring to deglaze the pan. Transfer to Crock-Pot, and add in the hot peppers, diced tomatoes, chicken and sausage. Cook on LOW for 5-6 hours.

Then add the rice, shrimp and parsley. Cook on HIGH for 1 hour (until rice is tender and all liquid is absorbed).

Again, I don't eat the sausage.

Snacks

I don't know about you, but I need to eat snacks, especially at night. But I stay away from everything fried, salty or fatty.

Here are some of the things that work for me:

Popcorn—I use an air popper (no oil or butter). As the popcorn comes out, I spray it lightly with butter-flavored cooking spray, and sprinkle parmigiano cheese on it.

Fruit and yogurt. I dice the fruit—could be pears, apples, watermelon, cantaloupe, honeydew, oranges, blueberries or any combination thereof—and stir it up in a bowl with fat-free vanilla yogurt.

"Unsalted" pretzels or "unsalted" potato chips (though I haven't actually eaten the chips in years; I try to stay away from everything fried). Once I got used to the taste of unsalted pretzels, I found them addictive.

Unsalted-tops Saltines, with reduced fat peanut butter.

Be creative. There's a lot more out there than potato chips, cookies or ice cream.

About the Authors

Stu Segal *is a voracious consumer of film and literature; he writes, rides motorcycles, juggles balls, clubs & knives, listens to rock 'n roll and plays drums. You can find him annually at the World Science Fiction Convention, the Westminster Kennel Club Show, rock concerts and motorcycle events, on the internet, and occasionally in the French Quarter.*

Stu was raised in Atlantic City, New Jersey. He went into banking as a coin wrapping clerk, and concluded his banking career 24 years later as vice president of a global bank, and on the Board of Directors of the New York Cash Exchange. He subsequently opened motorcycle dealerships selling Harley-Davidsons, Hondas and Triumphs. In 2012, he co-authored the popular music education book, "How to Read Drum Music".

He now lives just outside New York City, and can be contacted at stu.segal@ssegal.net

Dr. Ian J. Molk, M.D., F.A.C.C. *is board certified in both internal medicine and cardiology. He has been in private practice specializing exclusively in cardiology for nearly 30 years. He is also an assistant clinical professor of medicine at Robert Wood Johnson Medical School in New Jersey, where he is deeply involved in the education of residents.*

He was born and raised in Johannesburg, South Africa. After completing his M.D. at the University of Witwatersrand Medical School, he left for England then emigrated to the USA. He spent five years at SUNY at Stony Brook, New York, the first two doing anesthesia before switching specialties to internal medicine. He decided to specialize in cardiology and completed his cardiology fellowship at Stony Brook.

Dr. Molk loves practicing cardiology. He finds motivating and guiding his patients to improve their cardiac health, as well as keeping current on the latest advancements in the field, to be both challenging and personally rewarding. Dr. Molk's practice is in Edison, New Jersey.

Made in the USA
San Bernardino, CA
15 December 2013